Principles of Surgery Vivas for the MRCS

RUPEN DATTANI

RIDZUAN FAROUK

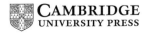

CAMBRIDGE
UNIVERSITY PRESS

CAMBRIDGE UNIVERSITY PRESS

Cambridge, New York, Melbourne, Madrid, Cape Town, Singapore, São Paulo

Cambridge University Press
The Edinburgh Building, Cambridge CB2 8RU, UK

Published in the United States of America by Cambridge University Press, New York

www.cambridge.org
Information on this title: www.cambridge.org/9780521699037

© Cambridge University Press 2007

First published 2007

Printed in the United Kingdom at the University Press, Cambridge

A catalogue record for this publication is available from the British Library

ISBN-13 978-0-521-69903-7 paperback

Principles of Surgery Vivas for the MRCS

WO18 DAT

2/10/08

14/4/09

29·4·09

7

Contents

Acknowledgements

I am eternally grateful to my family whose continual love, support and encouragement have helped me achieve all I have in life. I would like to dedicate this book to Sunny, a truly missed friend whose enthusiasm and love for life remain my constant source of inspiration.

R. D.

Abdominal Aortic Aneurysm (AAA)

Define an abdominal aortic aneurysm

It is an abnormal permanent localised dilatation of the aorta having at least a 50% increase in diameter compared with the expected normal diameter. It is usually regarded as a diameter >3 cm.

What is the aetiology of AAA?

- Hypertension
- Peripheral vascular disease
- Hyperlipidaemia
- Diabetes mellitus
- Increasing age
- Sex (M : F = 4 : 1)
- Family history

What are the clinical features of AAA?

- Asymptomatic (75%)
- Symptomatic:
  - pain: epigastric or back
  - rupture
  - distal embolus
  - fistula: aorto-caval; aorto-intestinal
  - systemic illness (inflammatory aneurysms)

How are AAAs diagnosed?

- Clinically: pulsatile expandable abdominal mass
- Ultrasound
- CT

What is the natural history of AAA?

The risk of rupture increases as aneurysm expands. Growth is usually at 10%/yr. The 5-year risk of rupture is 15% for aneurysms <4 cm, this increases to >75% for aneurysms >7 cm. Overall, only about 15% of all AAA ever rupture, the remainder die from unrelated causes. The overall mortality from a rupture is 80%–90%.

What is the role of screening in AAA?

Pilot schemes have shown that screening for asymptomatic AAA can reduce the rate of rupture by almost 50%. High risk patients, e.g. hypertensive males >65 could be targeted for such screening programmes. Patients with small aneurysms could undergo regular USS surveillance. A multicentre screening programme study is currently under way to determine the feasibility of a national screening programme.

Briefly describe the UK small aneurysm trial

This trial randomised 1090 asymptomatic infra-renal small aneurysms (4.0–5.5 cm) in patients aged between 60 and 76 to operate or be kept under regular ultrasound surveillance. There was no difference in mortality rates from early surgical repair compared with 6-monthly ultrasound surveillance. Annual rupture rate in this study was 1%. Surgical intervention was used when one of the following three criteria was met.

- Rate of expansion >1 cm/yr
- Aneurysm diameter expansion >5.5 cm
- Aneurysm became symptomatic or tender on palpation

What are the indications for surgery in patients with AAA?

Emergency repair:
- Rupture
- Rapidly expanding (>1 cm/yr) aneurysm that is symptomatic or clinically tender

Elective repair:
- Aneurysms >5.5 cm in diameter
- Symptomatic aneurysm
- Rate of expansion >1 cm/yr that is asymptomatic and non-tender

How should patients with smaller aneurysms be managed?
- Aneurysm <4 cm: yearly USS surveillance
- Aneurysm 4–5.5 cm: 6-monthly USS surveillance

What are the surgical options in the treatment of AAAs?
- Endoluminal repair: trans-femoral or trans-iliac placement of prosthetic graft under fluoroscopic guidance. The three main types of graft are: aorto–aorto, aortobi–iliac and aortouni–iliac with a femoral–femoral crossover. Requires CT or IADSA to evaluate the morphology of the aneurysm prior to the procedure. About 1–1.5 cm of healthy aorta distal to the renal arteries and 1 cm in the common iliac arteries required for sufficient clearance, therefore only about 40% of aneurysms suitable for this type of repair. Successful stenting associated with reduced aneurysm expansion. Patients require post-procedure CT to detect for endoleaks, which can cause ruptures. Other complications include graft migration and displacement, graft occlusion, infection, embolisation and graft kinking.
- Open repair: durable synthetic materials, e.g. Dacron® used for repair. Mortality rate between 2% and 5% and rises to 10% for patients with associated co-morbidity. Specific complications include:
  - immediate: bleeding, embolism, arterial thrombosis
  - early: acute renal failure, CVA, MI, mesenteric infarction, spinal cord ischaemia
  - late: graft infection, false aneurysm, aorto-enteric fistula

■ Abdominal Pain

What are the common causes of acute abdominal pain?
- Non-specific abdominal pain
- Appendicitis
- Intestinal obstruction
- Biliary tract disease: cholelithiasis, choledocholithiasis, calculus, cholecystitis, ascending cholangitis and gallstone ileus
- Diverticular disease: painful diverticula, diverticulitis, perforated diverticula
- Peptic ulcer disease
- Pancreatitis
- Constipation
- Inflammatory bowel disease
- Irritable bowel syndrome
- Bacterial/viral gastroenteritis
- Irritable bowel syndrome
- Abdominal aortic aneurysm: seen mainly in elderly patients
- Malignancy: high incidence in elderly
- Mesenteric ischemia
- Urological causes: UTI, calculi, testicular torsion
- Medical cause:
  - myocardial infarction
  - pneumonia
- Gynaecological causes of abdominal pain
  - ectopic pregnancy
  - pelvic inflammatory disease
  - endometriosis
  - ruptured ovarian cyst

Which investigations may be useful in the diagnosis of abdominal pain/masses?

- CXR: helpful in excluding pneumonia and free intraperitoneal air under the diaphragm in patients with ruptured viscus
- AXR: it is of limited use in the young patient but may show air within an abscess or as a result of intestinal obstruction or perforation; calcium deposition may be seen in chronic pancreatitis and calculi (renal or biliary); late findings of mesenteric ischaemia occasionally observed (i.e. pneumatosis intestinalis)
- Ultrasound: does not involve radiation but limitations to use include: obesity, poor images in the presence of gas and is operator dependent. Can be used to:
  - identify nature of lesion: cystic or solid
  - determine vascularity of a mass (Doppler)
  - guide biopsy of a mass
  - identify liver metastases
- CT: significant radiation but rapid results, not operator dependent and not influenced by presence of gas. Uses include:
  - differentiating cysts from abscesses
  - staging of cancers
  - diagnosing intra-abdominal lymphadenopathy
  - high sensitivity for diverticulitis
  - in stable patients with suspected AAA
  - CT with angiography: for suspected mesenteric ischaemia
- Double contrast barium enema: indicated if a mass is thought to arise from the large bowel, e.g. cancers, polyps, diverticular disease, inflammatory bowel disease ('cobblestoning' or skip lesions)
- Instant enema: indicated for acute large bowel obstruction

- Barium meal and small bowel enema: for masses arising from the stomach or small bowel
- IVU: for some urological causes of abdominal pain
- Radioisotope imaging: used when other modalities have not confirmed diagnosis.
- MRI: used in pelvic masses and liver lesions

■ Abscesses

What is an abscess?
An abscess is a loculated or localised collection of pus surrounded by granulation tissue. It usually contains bacteria or other pathogens, inflammatory cells, necrotic tissue and protein exudates. It can be superficial (e.g. pilonidal, breast) or deep (e.g. diverticular, subphrenic).

What are the clinical features of an abscess?
- Localised inflammation
- 'Pointing' (the tracking of an abscess to an external surface)
- Discharge of pus (purulent) or pus mixed with blood (haemopurulent)
- On examination:
  - locally: swelling, central tenderness, fluctuant mass
  - generally: pyrexia, tachycardia, sepsis

Which group of patients are at particular risk of abscess formation?
- Immunocompromised patients
- Sickle cell
- Peripheral vascular disease
- Inflammatory bowel disease
- Severe trauma

What is the role of antibiotics in the treatment of abscesses?
Abscess cavities are impervious to antibiotics and in fact prolonged antibiotic treatment can result in a chronic

inflammatory mass (an 'antibioma'). All abscesses should therefore be drained.

How can abscesses be drained?

- Aspiration: abscesses filled with fluid can be aspirated with a large bore needle and the process repeated if necessary. This method should only be used if there is no continuing cause found
- Open drainage: superficial abscesses can usually be drained through a cruciate incision; the pus sent for microbiology; loculi broken down and necrotic tissue excised. The wound should be left open and packed with an appropriate dressing
- Percutaneous drainage: deep abscess can be drained by fluoroscopic, ultrasound or CT guided aspiration. A tube can be left *in situ* to allow drainage of fluid

■ Alcohol and Surgery

Which surgical specialities might be involved in the management of patients with excessive alcohol consumption?

- General surgery:
  - Mallory–Weiss tear
  - oesophageal varices
  - oesophageal carcinoma
  - gastritis, gastric erosions and ulcers
  - gastric carcinoma
  - acute and chronic pancreatitis
  - pancreatic carcinoma
  - liver cirrhosis
  - hepatomegaly
  - splenomegaly, hypersplenism
  - hepatocellular carcinoma
- Trauma and orthopaedics:
  - road traffic accidents
  - fragility fractures: altered calcium metabolism causes osteoporosis thus increasing the risk of fractures
  - alcoholic myopathy: characterised by painful and swollen muscles
- ENT:
  - laryngeal carcinoma
  - pharyngeal carcinoma
- Neurosurgery:
  - head injury with intracranial bleeding
- Urology:
  - impotence
  - testicular atrophy

- Obstetrics and Gynaecology:
  - irregular menses
  - fetal alcohol syndrome

What are the potential problems of surgery in patients with excessive alcohol consumption?

Pre-operatively:

- Obtaining a detailed history may be difficult due to memory loss, confabulations, cerebellar degeneration, Korsakov's psychosis or Wernicke's encephalopathy
- Nutritional deficiencies are common even in well-nourished alcoholics:
  - vitamins: thiamine, folate, pyridoxine, nicotinic acid, vitamin A
  - electrolyte imbalance: low serum levels of potassium, magnesium, zinc, calcium, phosphorus
- Patients are more likely to have alcohol-induced medical problems:
  - cardiovascular: hypertension, arrhythmias (especially atrial fibrillation), cardiomyopathy, heart failure, mural thrombus formation, cerebrovascular accidents
  - respiratory: blood flow to the lungs may be impeded in chronic alcoholics with cirrhosis of the liver who can have up to 30% of their cardiac output shunting right to left, thereby decreasing oxygenation; alcoholics frequently have pulmonary aspiration due to central nervous system depression when intoxicated, leading to aspiration pneumonitis
  - renal: alcohol exerts a diuretic effect by inhibiting the secretion of ADH; serum sodium may be increased and potassium decreased in chronic alcoholics with increased total body water content
  - endocrine: glucose intolerance, transient hypoglycaemia

- haematological: macrocytic anaemia, thrombocytopenia, prolonged prothrombin time and partial thromboplastin time
- Drug interactions:
  - acceleration of hepatic microsomal metabolism of certain drugs, e.g. warfarin, hypnotic agents, antidepressants, antihistamines and hypoglycaemic drugs
  - liver pathology may depress metabolism and slow the clearance of drugs from the liver, thus increasing the half-life of certain drugs administered to the patient

Operatively:
- Excessive bleeding due to:
  - altered liver production of clotting factors II, V, VII, X and XIII
  - portal hypertension
  - decreased platelet aggregation
  - inhibited thromboxane A2 production, which is required for clotting

Post-operatively: alcoholics have a higher incidence of:
- pulmonary infection: alcohol inhibits ciliary activity, macrophage mobilisation and surfactant production
- wound infections due to decreased production of white blood cells and reduced granulocyte mobility
- anastomotic leakages

What is alcohol withdrawal syndrome?

Alcohol withdrawal syndrome occurs when patients who have ethanol-induced cellular tolerance to alcohol stop drinking. The symptoms are due to the sudden withdrawal of the CNS depressant effects of alcohol and can range from a mild hangover effect to life-threatening seizures. Clinical features of withdrawal include a tremor of the hands, autonomic nervous system dysfunction (e.g. increases in pulse, respiratory rate, temperature and blood pressure, insomnia and nightmares, anxiety or panic attacks) and GI disturbance. Symptoms commence within 0 to 5 hours of reducing alcohol intake, peak in intensity on day 2 or 3 and usually begin to improve by the fourth or fifth day of withdrawal. About 5% of patients in withdrawal exhibit severe symptoms, e.g. delirium tremens (a confusional state accompanied with hallucinations) or generalised seizures.

Prevention of alcohol withdrawal is important in the patient undergoing surgery and in the post-operative period. Benzodiazepines (e.g. Chlordiazepozide or diazepam), alpha-agonists and carbamazepine have been shown to decrease the incidence of withdrawal including seizures. Beta blockers can be added to prevent autonomic dysfunction.

A   Alcohol and Surgery

■ Amputation

What are the main indications for amputation surgery?
3 **Ds**: dead, deadly or disabled.
- Dead (gangrene)
  - vascular disease (arterial or venous)
  - diabetes mellitus
  - infection
- Deadly (tumour)
- Disabled
  - trauma
  - congenital deformity

Dead
Deadly
Disabled

What are the contraindications?
- Joint contractures affecting the hip and/or knees
- Severe osteoarthritis
- Spasticity or paralysis of the lower limbs
- Sensory neuropathy affecting the skin of the future stump

How can amputations be classified?
- Major:
  - lower limb: hindquarter, hip disarticulation, above-knee, through knee, below-knee
  - upper limb: forequarter, shoulder disarticulation, upper arm, forearm
- Minor:
  - lower limb: toe, Ray, transmetatarsal, midfoot, ankle
  - upper limb: digit, Ray

What factors influence the level of amputation to be performed?

- Viability of soft tissues
- Vascular viability: this can be assessed clinically (skin colour, atrophic changes, temperature) or using specific investigations, i.e. Doppler scans, transcutaneous P_{O_2} measurement or isotope measurement of skin blood flow
- Viability of underlying bone: X-rays should be taken in at least two planes
- Underlying pathology
- Functional requirement
- Ability of the patient to rehabilitate
- Comfort
- Cosmetic appearance

What are the general principles of amputation surgery?

Pre-operative:

- Multidisciplinary approach with input from the surgeon, anaesthetist, physician in rehabilitation medicine, nursing staff, physiotherapists, occupational therapists, prosthetic specialists and psychologists
- Assessment of the level of amputation to be performed: comprises clinical assessment and adjunctive investigations
- Consider epidural analgesia pre-operatively (which can be continued to the post-operative period) as it significantly reduces post-operative phantom pain
- Antibiotic prophylaxis
- Avoid the use of tourniquets in vascular disease

Operative:

- The total length of the flap should be approximately one and a half times the diameter of the leg at the level of bone resection

- Blood vessels should be dissected and separately ligated to prevent the development of arteriovenous fistulas and aneurysms
- Nerves should be divided under tension and proximal to the bone section to avoid neuroma formation
- Remove any bony prominences around disarticulations
- Muscle (assess viability) should be used to cover the cut end of bones
- Avoid excessive soft tissue within the stump
- Tension-free closure
- Consider the use of a drain especially for major amputations

Post-operative:
- Strong analgesia is essential as these procedures are painful
- Early physiotherapy: to prevent flexion contractures, build muscle power, prevent stump oedema and to commence early mobilisation
- Use of early walking aids (prosthesis): allows the patient to stand and commence walking with the physiotherapist
- Support groups can be beneficial

What are the postoperative complications of amputation surgery?
- Early:
  - infection of the soft tissues
  - haematoma at stump site
  - wound breakdown
  - flexion contractures
  - DVT / PE
- Late:
  - phantom limb pain
  - causalgia

- infection (including osteomyelitis)
- ischaemia
- ulceration
- bone erosion through the skin

■ Anaemia and Surgery

Define anaemia
Hb concentration <14 g/dl in men and <12 g/dl in women.

What is the ideal perioperative haemoglobin concentration in anaemic patients undergoing surgery?
For optimal tissue oxygen delivery an Hb of 10–11g/dl is required.

Why might it be important to correct chronic anaemia prior to surgery?
- Anaemic patients have reduced capacity to compensate for intra-operative blood loss
- Anaemia reduces tissue oxygenation due to:
  - shifting of Hb dissociation curve to the right
  - reduction in plasma viscosity
  - local tissue acidosis
  - peripheral vasodilation

When should patients be transfused in the preoperative period?
There is not a single figure at which transfusion should be commenced. A decision to transfuse should be made by determining the minimal Hb concentration that will provide adequate tissue oxygenation for that individual.

How much will the haemoglobin concentration rise after transfusion of one unit of red cells?
In an average 70 kg adult, Hb concentration will rise by 1.1 g/dl.

What are the problems with preoperative allogenic blood transfusion?

- Elevation of Hb concentrations to 'normal' levels can worsen heart failure and cause cardiac failure
- Blood transfused immediately prior to surgery has reduced O_2 carrying capacity
- Pre-operative transfusion may induce immunosuppression
- Increased risk of post-operative infection especially in orthopaedic patients
- Increased risk of tumour recurrence and death
- Increased hospital stay

If transfusion is required when should it be given?

Ideally, it should be given at least 2 days before surgery.

What are the alternatives to allogenic blood transfusion?

- Drug therapy:
  - haematinics, i.e. ferrous sulphate or recombinant human erythropoietin (EPO) administered a few weeks prior to surgery can increase the red cell mass and haematocrit with a reduction in the need for intra-operative transfusion
  - anti-fibrinolytics (e.g. tranexamic acid) have proven to reduce blood loss during cardiac and liver transplantation surgery
- Pre-operative autologous blood donation (PAD): should be considered if there is a likelihood of at least 2 units of red cells being required for intraoperative transfusion. Average donation is 1 unit/wk therefore not suitable for emergency surgery
- Acute normovolaemic haemodilution: at the start of surgery blood is removed from the patient and the volume replaced with intravenous fluid. The collected blood can be

transfused at the end of surgery or as required intra-operatively

- Intra-operative cell salvage: batched or continuous processing of blood collected during surgery which can be transfused back into the patient

◼ Anastomoses

What are the basic principles in performing any gastrointestinal anastomoses?

Pre-operatively:

- Optimisation of any co-existing medical conditions
- Bowel preparation: to reduce intraoperative peritoneal contamination
- Nutritional supplementation
- Prophylactic antibiotics

Operatively:

- Adequate exposure
- Careful assessment of the extent of resection required:
  - ensure both ends of the bowel to be joined have a good vascularity
- Minimise risk of infection:
  - isolate the cut ends of bowel with antiseptic-soaked swabs
  - use of polythene wound protectors may help prevent contamination of wound edges
  - clean open ends of the bowel with antiseptic-soaked swabs
  - after instruments have been used for an anastomosis, they should not be used again, e.g. for wound closure
- Suturing during formation of an anastomosis should be such that:
  - the bowel is not rendered ischaemic (not too many sutures!)
  - the knots are not over-tightened
  - the sutures are equally spaced
  - the bowel edges are approximated and inverted

- Anastomoses should be:
  - tension free
  - watertight
  - free of foreign material
- At the end of the procedure ensure that:
  - the bowel is lying untwisted and without tension
  - there is an adequate lumen
  - any mesenteric defect is repaired
- Consider a proximal defunctioning stoma especially if a high risk of anastomotic leakage is anticipated. This is particularly relevant if a low, colo-rectal or colo-anal anastomosis has been performed. In such cases, formation of a loop ileostomy can be considered (integrity of anastomosis is confirmed with a contrast study, 6–8 weeks post-surgery, before the stoma is reversed)

Post-operatively:

- Anastomosis healing can be optimised by:
  - ensuring optimisation of the patient's general condition
  - preventing generalised hypoxia (this will cause tissue hypoxia)
  - preventing hypovolaemia (this will reduce splanchnic blood flow and in turn, will lead to anastomotic failure)
- After an oesophago-gastric or oesophago-jejunal anastomosis, many surgeons will perform water-soluble contrast studies prior to commencing oral intake
- Always be vigilant for signs of an anastomotic leak

What are the different techniques of performing a gastrointestinal anastomosis?

- Anastomoses can be fashioned in three ways:
  - end to end
  - end to side
  - side to side

- Hand sewn:
  - single-layered: strong submucosal layer with minimal damage to submucosal blood vessels; interrupted seromuscular absorbable suture
  - two-layered: serosal apposition and mucosal inversion; inner continuous and outer interrupted suture
- Stapled:
  - side-to-side anastomoses with linear staples
  - end-to-end anastomoses with circular devices

How do anastomoses heal?

- Lag phase (day 0–4): inflammatory phase; anastomoses have minimal strength
- Fibroplasia phase (day 4–14): immature collagen laid down; anastomoses still weak
- Maturation phase (after day 10): collagen remodels; anastomoses strengthen

Why do gastrointestinal anastomoses fail?

- Poor patient selection:
  - immunocompromised patients, e.g. malnutrition, corticosteroid therapy, jaundice, sepsis, uraemia
- Poor preparation of the intestine for the anastomosis:
  - bowel ends were of poor vascularity
  - there was distal obstruction
- Poor surgical technique:
  - bowel ends under tension during anastomoses
  - sutures not tied correctly or knots tied too tightly rendering the bowel ischaemic
  - mesenteric defects not repaired
  - peri-anastomotic haematoma formation
- Poor post-operative care:
  - hypoxia or hypotension leading to tissue ischaemia

What are the signs of anastomotic leakage?

- Intra-luminal contents in a drain
- Sepsis
- Peritonitis
- Fistula formation
- Unexplained pyrexia or elevated white blood count
- Prolonged ileus or a chest infection developing at a later than usual stage
- Progress is slower than expected

How does vascular anastomosis differ from gastrointestinal anastomosis?

In order to appose the inner endothelial layers, vascular anastomosis must be performed by eversion and not inversion as is the case for intestinal anastomosis. Failure to do this will allow clots to form at the anastomosis and occlude the lumen. For very small vessels, eversion is not possible and so the anastomosis is performed such that the ends are united, edge-to-edge using a series of interrupted sutures.

■ Antibiotic Prophylaxis

What is the aim of antibiotic prophylaxis?
It is to prevent bacteria from multiplying without altering the normal tissue flora.

What are the indications for antibiotic prophylaxis?
General indications:
- when a procedure commonly leads to infection, e.g. colectomy
- when antibiotic prophylaxis has been shown to be of proven value in reducing post-operative infections from endogenous sources
- when results of infection would be devastating despite the low risk of occurrence, e.g. insertion of metallic prosthesis
- immunocompromised patients
- urinary catheterisation in patients with prosthetic joint implants or heart valves
- removal of a urinary catheter in all patients
- surgery in patients with valvular heart disease or prosthetic heart valves to prevent endocarditis

Urological surgery in patients:
- requiring instrumentation of the upper urinary tract
- with known urinary tract infection
- with potentially infected urine (urinary calculi disease or catheterised patients) who are at greater risk of infection
- with urinary tract infection and who are known to have valvular heart disease or prosthetic heart valves
- at higher risk of systemic infection, e.g. diabetics, patients with congenital cardiac disorders, patients with a cardiac pacemaker or metallic orthopaedic implants

When and how should antibiotic prophylaxis be administered?

Intravenously, usually 1 h before surgery or at induction of anaesthesia and at least 5 minutes before inflation of a tourniquet. Second dose should be given if surgery lasts >4 h or if there is significant blood loss or haemodilution, to maintain adequate tissue levels. It can be given as a single dose (if post-operative infection rate is 3%–6%) or multiple doses (if post-operative infection rate > 6%).

What factors influence the choice of antibiotic used?

All hospitals should have antibiotic prophylaxis protocols in place that must be reviewed and updated regularly. Factors that influence the choice of antibiotic used are:

- site of surgery: different body sites have different bacterial flora
- sensitivity to encountered organisms
- side effects
- geographical resistance to organisms

■ Anticoagulation Therapy and Surgery

When is it safe to perform surgery in patients on warfarin?

Surgery is normally safe when the INR is less than 1.2.

How should patients on warfarin be managed prior to elective surgery?

- Warfarin should be stopped 4–5 days before surgery
- Intravenous heparin infusion commenced once the INR is <2 or 24 hours after the last dose of warfarin for patients in whom anticoagulation is critical (e.g. patients with mechanical heart valves)
- APTT measured regularly and be kept in the therapeutic range (2–3)
- Heparin should be stopped 6 hours before surgery, at which time the APTT ratio should be <1.5
- Immediately after surgery, heparin infusion should be restarted and warfarin commenced once the patient is eating normally. Heparin is stopped once the INR is >2

How should patients on warfarin be managed during emergency surgery?

- Pre-operatively, 10 mg intravenous phytomenadione (vitamin K$_1$) is given followed by 15 ml/kg fresh frozen plasma
- Coagulation profile should be measured during surgery and FFP infusion repeated

What is the problem with phytomenadione (vitamin K$_1$) treatment?

Patients may be resistant to re-warfarinisation for up to 4 weeks following administration

Is it important to measure the activity of low molecular weight heparin treatment (LMWH)?

No. Although LMWH activity can be assessed by measuring Factor Xa levels, this is not required as the bioavailability of these drugs is more predictable than that of unfractionated heparin. LMWH should be stopped 12 hours before surgery.

What is the effect of antiplatelet agents on surgery?

Antiplatelet agents such as aspirin and dipyridamole will lead to prolonged bleeding which can be seen up to 2 weeks after cessation of treatment. In some types of surgery, i.e. neurosurgery, these agents are stopped routinely prior to operation.

■ Assessment for Fitness for Anaesthesia

What is the single most important factor which influences post-operative mortality rates?

The National Confidential Enquiry into Perioperative Death (NCEPOD) identified sub-optimal pre-operative preparation of patients as the leading factor.

What are the most common reasons for cancellation of an operation on the day of surgery?

- Onset of new medical condition
- Insufficient optimisation of co-existing conditions
- Inadequate investigations of co-existing conditions
- Lack of critical care beds (less common than above three factors)

How can cancellation rates be reduced?

- Pre-operative assessment clinics run by anaesthetists to deal with patients with complicated medical histories
- Early referral to medical specialists to assess if the patient's condition can be optimised prior to surgery

Which medical conditions are commonly sub-optimally controlled prior to surgery?

- Cardiac
- Respiratory
- Renal failure

What is the ASA grading system?

The American Society of Anesthesiologists (ASA) grade is the most commonly used grading system, which accurately predicts morbidity and mortality associated with anaesthesia and surgery.

ASA Grade	Definition	Mortality (%)
I	Normal healthy individual	0.05
II	Mild systemic disease with no functional limitation	0.4
III	Severe systemic disease with functional limitation	4.5
IV	Severe systemic disease which is a constant threat to life	25
V	Moribund patient, not expected to survive 24 hours with or without surgery	50

■ Atelectasis

Why should doctors and surgeons know something about atelectasis?

Atelectasis is a common cause of post-operative pyrexia. It usually manifests about 48 hours post-surgery.

What is the mechanism causing atelectasis?

An enhanced quantity of bronchial secretions combined with an increased viscosity of the secretions results in difficulty in coughing. This, combined with an increased work of breathing and impaired gas exchange, will predispose to the collapse of a group of alveoli, a small lobule or rarely the whole lung and ultimately cause chest infections.

Which group of patients are particularly susceptible to severe atelectasis?

- Those with co-existing respiratory disease
- Smokers
- Obese

How can it be prevented?

- Pre-operative patient education about postoperative respiratory exercises
- Early mobilisation
- Frequent changes of position
- Encouragement to cough

What are the other symptoms and signs?

- Breathlessness
- Tachypnoea

- Hypoxia
- Tachycardia
- Reduced air entry and breath sounds on auscultation
- CXR shows consolidation and/or collapse

What is its management?
- Adequate oxygenation and fluid resuscitation
- Pain relief to allow patient to cough without discomfort
- Chest physiotherapy to remove secretions
- Nebulised saline with or without bronchodilators
- Antibiotics should only be given for super-imposed infections
- Mucolytic agents, tracheal suction or fibreoptic bronchoscopy occasionally required to extract mucus plugs

List the other causes of post-operative hypoxia
- Hypoventilation
- Bronchospasm
- Pneumothorax
- Pulmonary embolism
- Pneumonia
- Pulmonary oedema

Biopsy and Cytological Sampling

What is the difference between biopsy and cytology?

A biopsy is the process by which tissue is obtained for microscopic or other investigation. Diagnosis of diseases based on examination of individual cells and small clusters of cells is called cytology or cytopathology. Biopsy may be diagnostic or therapeutic, whilst cytology tests may be used for diagnosis or for screening.

What are the advantages and disadvantages of these techniques?

A cytology specimen is usually easier to obtain, causes minimal discomfort to the patient, is less likely to result in serious complications, and is cheaper than a tissue biopsy. Although, in many clinical situations, the accuracy of cytology and biopsy is the same, in some situations a biopsy result is more accurate, e.g. in the diagnosis of a follicular thyroid carcinoma. The other advantages of a biopsy are that it allows assessment of tumour invasion and in some cases an excisional biopsy may be the only treatment required.

Describe the different forms of biopsy techniques

- Fine Needle Aspiration (FNA): the least invasive of the biopsy techniques and one of the first-line diagnostic procedures in the evaluation of a palpable breast mass. The procedure has the capability of being both therapeutic and diagnostic, e.g. during aspiration of a breast cyst the aspirate is often green tinged and serous (diagnostic), and aspiration should collapse the cystic cavity (therapeutic)

- Core needle biopsy (CNB): involves removal of a core of deep tissue usually using a Trucutt needle. Samples obtained with CNB are often large enough to provide detailed histological and architectural information including the type and grade of the tumour, its invasiveness, as well as hormone receptor status. This is an advantage over FNA, particularly with patients who have large masses suggestive of cancer

- Shave biopsy: a scalpel or razor blade is used to shave off a thin layer of the lesion parallel to the skin. Shave biopsies will normally provide information about only the epidermis and high dermis. It is therefore indicated in dermatoses characteristically localised in these regions, such as keratoses, plane warts and benign pigmented lesions. In such cases it may be both diagnostic and curative. The shave biopsy may also be used to sample tumours such as basal and squamous cell carcinoma

- Punch biopsy: a small cylindrical punch is screwed into the lesion through the full thickness of the skin and a plug of tissue is removed. It is a fast, easy and inexpensive method for producing a cylinder of tissue from the skin surface to the underlying subcutaneous fat. It may be used to sample tumours and yields more information about depth of invasion than the shave biopsy

- Scissors biopsy: scissors are used to snip off superficial skin growths and lesions that grow from a stem or column of tissue. Such growths are sometimes seen on the eyelids or neck

- Excision biopsy: the most invasive form of biopsy in which the entire lesion is excised. It is typically reserved for suspicious lesions after lesser invasive approaches have been tried, or when a benign mass is being removed. It is usually performed under general anaesthesia. This technique can have disadvantages, e.g. if a tumour is particularly invasive and a margin of excision is not achieved, then further surgery will be required. Furthermore, neoplastic cells at the tumour margin are most likely to be actively dividing, and debulking a mass may leave the most malignant cells behind

- Incisional or wedge biopsy: in essence, this technique is similar to a small fusiform excision, but by definition takes only part of the lesion, as opposed to an excisional biopsy, which removes the entire lesion. It is used to evaluate diffuse/generalised skin diseases or to identify a tumour before attempting its total removal. In either situation a minimum of three samples should be collected in an attempt to obtain representative changes
- Endoscopic/arthroscopic biopsy: the endoscope or arthroscope can be used to view suspicious areas in the gastrointestinal tract, genitourinary tract, the respiratory tract or any joint. Advantages include the opportunity to see the lesion directly and the ability to take a tissue sample through the scope for further analysis

How are tissues sampled for cytology?

- Fine needle aspiration (FNA): e.g. for thyroid lesions or lymph nodes
- Body cavity fluids: urine, sputum, CSF, pleural fluid, pericardial fluid, ascitic fluid can all be assessed for cytology
- Exfoliative: cells are scraped from the organ or tissue being tested, e.g. the *Pap test* for the cervix
- Brush: cells are brushed from the organ or tissue being tested, e.g. the oesophagus, stomach, bronchi or mouth

What happens to biopsy and cytology specimens after they are removed from the patient?

The specimen is placed in a container with preservative (usually formalin) and taken to the pathology laboratory where gross examination will determine which parts of the large biopsy are the most critical to study for microscopy. The tissue is then placed into a mould with hot paraffin wax and the embedded tissue cut into very thin slices. These thin slices are placed on glass slides and dipped into a series of stains. For most biopsy specimens, routine processing as described above is all that is technically required.

What is a frozen section examination?

Sometimes, information about a tissue sample is needed during surgery, so that decisions can be made about the immediate surgical treatment. When a frozen section examination is performed, fresh tissue is sent from the operating room directly to the pathologist. The fresh tissue is grossly examined and instead of processing the tissue in wax blocks, it is quickly frozen in a special solution and then thinly sectioned, quickly stained and examined under the microscope. This usually takes 10 to 20 minutes. Although the frozen sections usually do not display features of the tissue as clearly as sections of tissue embedded in wax, they are usually clear enough to evaluate whether an adequate margin of excision of a tumour has been achieved.

Bone Grafts

What do the terms osteogenesis, osteoinduction and osteoconduction mean?

These are the three unique properties that are essential for successful healing and incorporation of bone grafts

Osteogenesis: ability of bone to self-generate new bone formation

Osteoinduction: ability of bone to recruit mesenchymal stem cells from the surrounding host, which then differentiate into new bone

Osteoconduction: process of ingrowth of capillaries, perivascular tissue and osteoprogenitor cells from the host bed into graft structure. Graft functions as a scaffold for ingrowth of new bone

List the use of bone grafts

They are used to replenish bone loss that occurs with:
- loosening of prosthesis, e.g. in revision arthroplasty
- trauma
- tumours

Classify bone grafts

- Autografts: bone harvested from the patient's own skeleton
- Allografts: bone harvested from another individual (dead or alive)
- Xenografts: bone harvested from another species

What are the common donor sites for allografts?

- Iliac crests
- Femoral heads from patients undergoing hip arthroplasty
- Fibula (mainly as vascularised grafts)

What are the advantages and limitations with the use of autografts?

Autografts are considered the gold standard of bone transplantation because they posses all the three properties of osteogenesis, osteoinduction and osteoconduction that are essential for successful healing and incorporation of bone grafts. Limitations include:

- only restricted amount of bone can be acquired by this technique and this is usually insufficient to fill large defects that are associated with loosening
- harvesting the graft from patient's own skeleton can compromise normal skeletal architecture and mechanical integrity of donor sites
- donor site complications and morbidity can result in increased patient recovery time, disability and chronic pain

Where are allografts obtained from?

- Femoral heads of other patients undergoing hip replacements
- Femurs or tibias harvested from fresh cadavers

What are the limitations with the use of allografts?

- They are mainly osteoconductive, have limited osteoinductive properties and lack osteogenesis
- Bacterial contamination
- Potential transmission of pathogens such as hepatitis B, hepatitis C and HIV
- Higher incidence of failure rates compared with autografts
- Demands for cancellous allografts may outstrip supply in the future

Are xenografts commonly used in clinical practice?

No. Although xenografts are available commercially, they are rarely used due to possible risk of transmitting zoonotic diseases and the lack of evidence supporting their ability to form living bone

What are the alternatives to bone grafts?

- Demineralised bone matrix: formed from autologous bone extracts consisting of non-collagenase proteins, bone growth factors and collagen
- Bone graft substitute materials made from:
  - ceramics, e.g. hydroxyapatite, tricalcium phosphate
  - bioactive glasses
  - collagen
- Bone morphogenic proteins
- Mesenchymal stem cells

■ Breast Cancer

What are the risk factors for the development of breast cancer?

- Female gender: female : male = 100 : 1
- Age: risk increases after the fifth decade
- Family history: risk if one affected first-degree relative is 1.5–2× higher; having two first-degree relatives affected (female or male) increases relative risk by more than 4–6 times; patient with a mother diagnosed when <60 years is at 2× increased risk; bilateral cancer in a first-degree relative may increase risk by more than 6 times.
- Age at birth of first child: if aged ≥30 years relative risk is 2× that of patients who gave birth when <20 years.
- Genetic predisposition: this risk factor accounts for <10% of breast cancers
  - Li–Fraumeni syndrome
  - Muir–Torre syndrome
  - Cowden disease
  - Peutz–Jeghers syndrome
  - *BRCA1* (17Q) mutations: accounts for almost half of high-risk familial inheritances of breast cancer
  - *BRCA2* (13Q) mutations
  - ataxia–telangiectasia
- Non-invasive carcinoma: ductal carcinoma *in situ* (DCIS) or lobular carcinoma *in situ* (LCIS) on previous biopsy
- Benign proliferative changes with atypical hyperplasia
- Early menarche and late menopause: weakly associated

Describe the NHS breast cancer screening programme

- Nationally co-ordinated programme with >80 breast screening units across the UK, each inviting women aged 50 to 70 for 3-yearly mammograms
- Mammograms taken in two views: one from above (craniocaudal) and one into the armpit diagonally across the breast (mediolateral)
- If abnormality seen on mammogram, women are recalled for triple assessment (>50% of screen detected abnormalities shown to be non-malignant following triple assessment)
- Mammograms not as effective in pre-menopausal women because the density of breast tissue makes it more difficult to detect problems and also because the incidence of breast cancer is lower. The average age of the menopause in the UK is 50. As women go past the menopause, the glandular tissue in their breast 'involutes' and the breast tissue is made up increasingly of only fat which is clearer on the mammogram
- Saves over 1400 lives every year in England alone

How is breast cancer diagnosed?

Triple assessment:

- Clinical evaluation: obvious lump, size discrepancy, nipple inversion, skin dimpling, scaling, oedema (peau d'orange) unilateral nipple discharge
- Radiology: (USS <35 years old; mammography >35 years old)
- Histology (True cut needle biopsy) or cytology (FNA): cytology reported as: C1 = inadequate sample; C2 = benign; C3 = equivocal; C4 = suspicious of malignancy; C5 = malignant

How is breast cancer classified?

World Health Organisation classifies breast tumours by histological pattern.

- Epithelial:
  - non-invasive: ductal and lobular carcinoma in situ (DCIS / LCIS)
  - invasive: ductal, lobular, mucinous, papillary, medullary, Paget's disease
- Mixed connective tissue and epithelial: Phyllodes tumour, carcinosarcoma
- Miscellaneous: e.g. primary lymphoma

What do you understand by the terms level I, II and III axillary clearance?

- Level I: nodes lateral to pectoralis minor
- Level II: (central) nodes behind pectoralis minor
- Level III: (apical) nodes above pectoralis minor

What are the surgical options in the management of breast cancer?

- Ductal excision: can be performed for nipple discharge suggestive of malignancy (bloody or spontaneous clear discharge from a single duct) without an associated palpable or radiographic lesion
- Wide local excision or lumpectomy: performed for palpable lumps suggestive of malignancy on needle biopsy or benign/ inconclusive findings on needle biopsy in the presence of high clinical suspicion (i.e. large mass fixed to the chest wall, atypical epithelial hyperplasia)
- Quadrantectomy: removal of an entire breast quadrant
- Total or simple mastectomy: removal of breast parenchyma, including nipple-areolar complex, with no node dissection
- Modified radical mastectomy: resection of breast parenchyma and levels I and II axillary nodes
- Patey modified radical mastectomy: modified radial mastectomy with additional removal of level III nodes and resection of pectoralis minor muscle

- Radical (Halsted) mastectomy: removal of entire breast, all axillary nodes and the pectoralis minor and major muscles. Rarely needed but may be required to treat local recurrence or locally advanced carcinoma after adjuvant therapy
- Sub-cutaneous/skin-sparing mastectomy: subcutaneous excision of breast parenchymal tissue and the nipple–areolar complex with preservation of the skin envelope. This procedure is often performed prophylactically in healthy patients with strong risk factors

What do you understand by the term 'breast conserving surgery (BCS)'?

This term is used to describe lumpectomy, quadrantectomy or segmental mastectomy with or without axillary dissection and adjuvant radiation therapy. Tumours suitable for such surgery include: small single tumours in a large breast; tumours located peripherally; and tumours without local spread or extensive nodal involvement. For tumours that are suitable for breast conservation, there is no difference in local recurrence or overall survival when BCS + radiotherapy is compared to mastectomy.

What are the indications for mastectomy?
- Multifocal disease
- Extensive DCIS
- Male patients
- Tumours >3 cm in small-/moderate-sized breasts
- Patient choice
- Central tumour
- Salvage surgery

Which nerves are in danger of being injured during a mastectomy?
- Thoracodorsal nerve (injury causes weakness of latissimus dorsi)

- Long thoracic nerve (injury results in winged scapula on arm extension)
- Intercostobrachial nerve: often sacrificed in dissecting axillary nodes; transection results in numbness around the axilla and upper arm
- Lateral and medial pectoral nerves (injuries are rare)
- Brachial plexus

What do you understand by the term 'sentinel node'?

The sentinel lymph node is the first draining axillary lymph node from the breast. By detecting the presence or absence of tumour in this node, it may be possible to predict the status of the axilla and potentially avoid the morbidity associated with axillary node dissection. A blue dye or radiolabelled colloid can be injected into the primary tumour and used to localise the first draining lymph node.

What is the role of adjuvant chemotherapy in breast cancer?

- It can be given pre-operatively (neo-adjuvant) to downgrade or shrink large or locally advanced tumours, thus increasing the chance of breast-conserving surgery rather than a mastectomy
- Post-operatively: administration depends on various factors, e.g. age, menopausal status, nodal involvement and tumour grade
- Commonly used regimens are:
  - CMF: cyclophosphamide, methotrexate, 5-FU
  - FEC: epirubicin, cyclophosphamide and 5-FU
  - E-CMF: epirubicin, followed by CMF
  - AC: doxorubicin (adriamycin) and cyclophosphamide
  - MMM: methotrexate, mitozantrone and mitomycin
- Tamoxifen is effective for 5 years post-surgery with benefits seen in both pre- and post-menopausal women. The

greatest benefit is observed in ER (+) tumours; some benefit in ER (−) tumours

What are the options in breast reconstruction following a mastectomy?

- Tissue expanders: placed under the pectoralis major muscle; saline can be added to the expander (via a subcutaneous filport) at regular intervals
- Pedicled myocutaneous flaps: two commonly used flaps are:
  - latissimus dorsi flap based on thoracodorsal vessels
  - transverse rectus abdominis (TRAM) flap based on superior epigastric vessels
- Free tissue transfer
- Nipples can be reconstructed by:
  - tattooing
  - if the nipple from the removed breast is definitely cancer free, it can be attached to the reconstructed breast
  - prosthetic (stick-on) nipples
  - using skin of a similar tone, usually from the area surrounding the other nipple or the top of the inner thigh

What are the prognostic factors in breast cancer?

- Age: younger age at diagnosis has a poorer prognosis
- Tumour size: larger tumours have worse prognosis
- Lymph node status: as number of affected nodes increases survival decreases
- Metastases: distant metastases reduces survival rates
- Histological type: improved prognosis with tubular, mucinous, papillary and micro-invasive tumours
- Histological grade: higher grades worsen prognosis
- Lymphatic/vascular invasion: increases risk of short-term systemic relapse
- Hormone and growth factor receptors status

- ER (+) tumours respond well to selective oestrogen receptor modulators, e.g. tamoxifen; conversely ER(−) tumours have improved response to chemotherapy and minimal benefit from tamoxifen
  - Her-2/neu protein expression is associated with increased incidence of recurrence and shortened overall survival
- Oncogenes: tumours that express C-erb-B2 oncogene are likely to be resistant to CMF chemotherapy and hormonal therapy

■ Burns

How can burns be classified?
- By depth:
  - first-degree: epidermis partially destroyed; basal membrane intact
  - second-degree (superficial): basal membrane partially destroyed
  - second-degree (deep): basal membrane totally destroyed; dermis partially damaged; epidermal cells still present around hair follicles
  - third-degree: epidermis and dermis totally destroyed; subcutaneous tissue damage; deeper tissues and organs may be affected
- By cause:
  - heat
  - electricity
  - radiation
  - chemical
  - inhalation

Describe the physiological processes that occur following a burn
- Cardiovascular:
  - hypovolaemia secondary to increased microvascular permeability and interstitial oedema
  - up to 50% reduction in cardiac output due to decrease in plasma volume
- Respiratory:
  - hypoxia due to hypovolaemic shock and increased oxygen consumption

- in inhalation injuries: airway oedema and obstruction, bronchospasm, reduced compliance and increased lung lymph production
- Metabolic: increase in metabolic rate and metabolic requirement

How can the severity of a burn be assessed?
- Rule of nines in adults (9% for head and neck, each arm, each leg; 2 × 9% for back of trunk and front of trunk; 1% for perineum)
- Lund–Browder chart in children (similar to the rule of nines chart but takes into account the relatively larger head and smaller legs in children)

How can partial and full thickness burns be distinguished clinically?

	Partial thickness	Full thickness
Colour	Red	White
Blanching	Yes	No
Sensation present	Yes	No
Light touch	Painful	Not painful
Hair preserved	Yes	No
Blistering	Prominent; some slough	Slight; lots of slough

Describe the immediate management of burns
- Ensure adequate airway: high flow O_2; intubation if laryngeal oedema suspected
- Remove the source of the burn: cut off clothes; remove any chemical debris and flood the affected area with cold water if there is evidence of heat transfer

- iv fluid replacement for burns >15% of skin area (or >10% in children or elderly). Fluid replacement can be calculated according to the formula:
- [weight (kg) ×% burn area] / 2. The calculated volume is given every 4 h for first 12 hours, every 6 h for the next 12 hours and then 12-hourly for the next 12 hours
- Adequate iv analgesia
- Monitor pulse, BP, SaO_2, temp and GCS
- Assess burn depth and cover with sterile covers, dry dressings or cling film
- Escharotomy for extensive chest burns which may cause respiratory compromise
- Nutritional support for burns >20% of skin area

What are the complications of burns and how are they treated?

• CVS: hypovolaemia, reduced cardiac output	iv fluids
• RS: ARDS, pneumonitis	O_2, CPAP, PEEP
• GIT: Curling's ulcers, paralytic ileus	H_2 antagonists, NG tube
• Renal: acute renal failure	Fluids, mannitol, dialysis
• CNS: seizures(especially in children)	Anticonvulsants
• Haematological: DIC	heparin, FFP
• Infection, sepsis and SIRS	antibiotics

What are the prognostic factors in outcome of burns?

Dependent on three factors: burns >40% surface area, age >60 years and presence of inhalational injury. Mortality rates are 0.3% with no risk factors, 3% with one factor present, 33% with two factors present and 87% with three factors present.

How should smoke inhalation be managed?

Investigations:

- Arterial blood gases and carboxyhaemoglobin levels
- Chest X-ray
- Fibreoptic bronchoscopy

Treatment:

- Consider early intubation (before oedema of upper airways makes this difficult)
- Ventilatory support
- High concentration O_2
- Hyperbaric O_2 therapy if carboxyhaemoglobin $>15\%$
- Nebulised bronchodilators (for wheezing)
- Chest physiotherapy
- Transfer to burns centre for major burns

Cancer Treatment I: Surgery

What is the role of surgery in the treatment of cancer?

- Diagnostic: advances in diagnostic imaging, cytology and interpretation of core biopsies have reduced the need for open biopsies and diagnostic surgery; excision biopsies for accurate diagnosis of lymphoma are sometimes indicated
- Curative for:
  - primary tumours
  - metastasis
- Debulking: followed by chemotherapy can increase survival rates, e.g. ovarian carcinomas
- Reconstructive, e.g. breast reconstruction following a mastectomy
- Prophylactic for conditions that may result in cancer:
  - proctocolectomy for familial adenomatous polyposis
  - colectomy for hereditary non-polyposis colon
  - mastectomy for women with a family history of breast cancer
- Palliative:
  - relief of presenting symptoms
  - prevention of distressing symptoms caused by local progression, e.g. gastrointestinal obstruction
  - prophylactic internal fixation for bony metastasis

What are the principles of curative surgery for primary cancers?

There are extensive variations in the surgical management of different types of cancers. However, certain basic principles can be used in all curative surgery. These are:
Pre-operative:

- the cancer must have been detected early
- staging should be performed
- adjuvant therapy administered, if indicated
- counselling of patients by trained and experienced staff
- meticulous planning including appropriate blood and radiological investigations
- multidisciplinary approach with the team comprising surgeons, oncologists, pathologists, radiologists, specialist nurses and other allied health care professionals, e.g. physiotherapists and occupational therapists

Operative:
- macroscopic clearance is mandatory
- wide resection margins if microscopic spread is suspected

Post-operative:
- adjuvant chemo- or radiotherapy, if indicated
- regular follow-up of patients

Cancer Treatment II: Chemotherapy

Classify chemotherapeutic agents
- Cycle-specific: effective throughout the cell cycle, e.g. cisplatin, 5-Fluorouracil
- Phase-specific: effective during part of the cell cycle, e.g. methotrexate, vincristine

What are their modes of action?
- Prevent cell division by cross-linking DNA strands, e.g. cisplatin, chlorambucil
- Impede with purine or pyramidine synthesis, e.g. methotrexate, 5-Fluorouracil
- Prevent RNA production, e.g. doxorubicin, bleomycin
- Inhibit the metaphase (M phase) of mitosis, e.g. vincristine, vinblastine

Which tumours respond to chemotherapy?
- Potentially curable:
  - acute lymphoblastic leukaemia
  - Wilms' tumour
  - germ cell tumours
  - Hodgkin's disease
  - Non-Hodgkin's lymphoma
  - testicular tumours
- Substantial response to chemotherapy:
  - breast carcinoma
  - ovarian carcinoma
  - osteosarcoma
  - lymphoma

- Palliative: controls symptoms and increases lifespan in advanced disease
  - breast carcinoma
  - myeloma
  - bladder cancer
  - soft tissue carcinoma
  - small cell lung cancer

Which tumours do not generally respond to chemotherapy?

- Colorectal carcinoma
- Gastric carcinoma
- Pancreatic carcinoma
- Melanomas

What are the general side-effects of chemotherapeutic agents?

- Diarrhoea or constipation
- Nausea and vomiting
- Abdominal pain
- Bone marrow depression
- Rash
- Alopecia
- Mucositis
- Infertility

Cancer Treatment III: Radiotherapy

How does radiotherapy work?

The cell is radiosensitive in the M-phase of the cell cycle. Radiation damages DNA directly via production of free radicals or from cross-linkages and indirectly via damage to proteins, enzymes or cell membranes. Damaged DNA inhibits cell replication resulting in cell death which in turn, stimulates other cells to divide and enter the M-phase.

What is fractionation?

It is the repeated use of low dose radiation within a course of treatment. In this manner, a higher total dose of radiation can be given, whilst allowing normal tissues time to repair.

What is the role of radiotherapy in the treatment of tumours?

- Primary treatment in:
  - sensitive tumours
  - inoperable tumours
  - patients not fit for surgery
- Adjuvant therapy:
  - pre- or post-operatively
  - at site of potential metastasis
- Palliation:
  - for relief of symptoms from primary tumour or metastasis, e.g. spinal cord compression, venous obstruction, pain from bony metastases

List some tumours that respond to radiotherapy

- Seminomas
- Hodgkin's and non-Hodgkin's lymphomas
- Gliomas
- Anal carcinoma
- Thyroid cancers
- Sarcomas

Which tumours do not respond to radiotherapy?

- Melanomas
- Pancreatic cancers

List some complications of radiotherapy

- Oesophagitis
- Oligospermia
- Acute leukaemia
- Premature menopause

What is interstitial radiation therapy?

It is another method of delivering radiation whereby small quantities of radium salt are implanted into the patient usually for several hours at a time. It is mainly used for well-localised tumours, e.g. anal cancers, tongue cancers and in the use of brachytherapy for prostate cancer.

■ Cancer Treatment IV: Hormonal Therapy

Which tumours respond to hormonal therapy?
- Prostate cancer
- Breast cancer
- Thyroid carcinoma
- Endometrial carcinomas

What is the role of hormone treatment in prostate cancer?

It is based on medical or surgical androgen ablation. About 90% of androgens are produced in the testis and the rest in the adrenal glands. The modes of treatment are blockade of androgen production in the:

- Hypothalamus–pituitary axis:
  - analogues of LH releasing hormones, e.g. goserelin
  - stilboestrol
  - cyproterone acetate
  - prednisolone
- Adrenal gland:
  - ketoconazole
  - aminogluthetimide
- Prostate:
  - flutamide
  - cyproterone acetate
- Testis:
  - bilateral orchidectomy

What is the role of hormone treatment in breast cancer?

Hormone therapy is beneficial in breast cancers that are oestrogen receptor or progesterone receptor positive (about 50%–80% of breast cancers). Only 5%–10% of receptor negative tumours will respond to hormonal treatment. Treatment options include:

- Selective oestrogenic receptor modulators:
  - tamoxifen (non-steroidal anti-oestrogen)
  - raloxifene (benzothiophene-selective oestrogen receptor modulator)
  - fluvestrant (anti-oestrogenic steroid)
- Inhibition of peripheral oestrogen production (aromatase inhibitors)
  - steroids – formestane, exemastane
  - non-steroids – anastrozole
- Oophorectomy
  - medical – LH releasing hormone analogues, e.g. goserelin
  - radiotherapy
  - surgical
- Progestogens
  - megestrol acetate

■ Cancer Treatment V: Cryotherapy and Immunotherapy

What is cryotherapy?

It is the treatment of viable tissues with freezing.

How does it work?

Cells are damaged by:

- ice formation causing cell membrane disruption
- electrolyte imbalance caused by thawing
- ischaemia caused to small vessels causing cellular hypoxia

Which diseases can be treated with cryotherapy?

- Benign conditions:
  - vascular: telangiectases, haemangiomas
  - skin: warts, pyogenic granulomas, keratoses
  - haemorrhoids
  - cervical erosions
- Pre-malignant conditions:
  - leukoplakia
  - Bowen's disease
  - rectal polyps
- Malignant lesions:
  - superficial skin cancers, e.g. basal cell carcinoma
  - cervical carcinoma
  - palliative treatment in cancers of the oral cavity

List the advantages and disadvantages of its use

Advantages:

- causes minimal scarring

- cost effective
- simple to use and can be performed as day case
- avoids the use of anaesthesia

Disadvantages:

- samples obtained are not always amenable to histological analysis
- can cause blistering
- can be painful

In which cancers has immunotherapy been of some benefit?

Renal cancer:	Interleukin 2 Alpha interferon
Bladder cancer:	BCG vaccine (used intravesically)

What is the advantage of immunotherapy over chemotherapy?

Immunotherapy attacks only malignant cells and does not damage normal cells thereby preventing the side effects seen with chemotherapy.

◼ Cardiac Disease and Surgery

List the common cardiac diseases that may be present in patients undergoing surgery
- Arterial hypertension
- Ischaemic heart disease
- Valvular heart disease
- Heart failure

What investigations may be useful in these patients?
- Bloods:
  - correct anaemia if present
  - correct electrolyte imbalance (caused by many cardiac drugs)
- CXR
- Resting ECG
- Exercise ECG:
  - economical method of assessing coronary artery disease
  - of limited use in patients unable to exercise to required rate to allow assessment
- Thallium scintigraphy:
  - highly sensitive and specific in diagnosing coronary artery disease
- Echocardiogram:
  - assesses left ventricular function
- Coronary angiogram:
  - may be required in patients with severe coronary artery disease proceeding to angioplasty or stenting

Are there any ways of assessing perioperative cardiac risk?

Yes. Several indices exist that provide an assessment of perioperative cardiac risk such as the Goldman Multifactorial Cardiac Risk Index (CRI), the Eagle Low-Risk Index and the Revised Cardiac Risk Index. All these indices are based on the type of surgery to be performed, the patient's cardiac and medical history, clinical findings and ECG findings.

Define hypertension. Why is it important to treat hypertension prior to surgery?

It is sustained diastolic pressure greater than 110 mmHg. Patients with uncontrolled hypertension elicit an exaggerated response during surgery with greater cardiovascular instability. Ideally, all patients should be treated prior to surgery and younger patients investigated for secondary causes of hypertension.

What is the risk of perioperative myocardial infarction (MI) following a recent myocardial infarction?

Time since MI	Risk of repeat MI (%)
<3 weeks	80
3 weeks–3 months	10–20
3–6 months	5–10
>6 months	1–2

What is the mortality rate following a post-operative myocardial infarction?

50%–70%. Half of these are silent. Highest incidence is on the third post-operative day.

What types of surgery are associated with post-operative myocardial infarction?

- High risk (>5%)
  - major emergency surgery
  - vascular surgery
  - surgery with high blood loss
- Intermediate risk (1–5%)
  - head and neck surgery
  - orthopaedic surgery
  - abdominal and thoracic surgery
  - pelvic surgery
- Low risk (<1%)
  - minor surgery
  - breast surgery
  - eye surgery

Which valvular heart disease poses the greatest problem with surgery?

Ideally, all patients with murmurs should have pre-operative echocardiography to assess the severity of the disease. The most significant disorder is aortic stenosis as it is associated with a low cardiac output. Anaesthesia in these patients causes hypotension which is poorly tolerated and does not respond to fluid filling.

Why is it imperative to treat cardiac failure prior to surgery?

Uncontrolled cardiac failure can result in acute heart failure, arrhythmias and high mortality rates following anaesthesia and surgery. Echocardiography can provide useful information regarding ventricular function. Left ventricular ejection fraction of <30% is associated with a high mortality rate.

▪ Carotid Artery Disease

What is the clinical presentation of carotid artery stenosis?

- Amaurosis fugax
- Transient ischaemic attack (TIA)
- Reversible intermittent neurological deficit (RIND)
- Evolving CVA
- Completed CVA
- Asymptomatic bruit

How can stenosis be assessed?

- Clinically: carotid bruit – can be unreliable in assessing the severity of stenosis and may be absent in severe stenosis
- Duplex ultrasound: main investigation used in most hospitals
- CT: detects small haemorrhages but not infarcts
- MRI: good for assessing small infarcts
- CT or MRI angiography: non-invasive technique without the risks associated with carotid angiography; limited availability is a problem
- Carotid angiography: allows assessment of the degree of stenosis and can give indication of any intracranial vascular disease; about 1% risk of CVA and 4% risk of inducing further neurological damage
- Transcranial doppler: can be used to test for cerebral reserve

What is the non-operative treatment of carotid artery disease?

- Modify risk factors: stop smoking, tight diabetic control
- Treat causative factors, e.g. hypertension, DM

- Prophylactic aspirin (combination with dipyridamole is no more effective than aspirin alone)

What are the indications for surgery?

For symptomatic patients (TIAs, amaurosis fugax, recovered stroke), clinical practice is based on the results of two large trials, the North American Symptomatic Carotid Endarterectomy Trial (NASCET) and the European Carotid Surgery trial (ECST) which concluded:
- there is benefit from surgery in patients with stenoses of 70%–99%, with up to 22% reduction in stroke 3 years after surgery
- no benefit from surgery in those with <70% stenoses
- peri-operative risk of stroke or death was 5.8% in NASCET and 7.5% in ECST
- angina and hypertension should be well controlled pre-operatively
- no benefit from surgery if patient selection is poor or complication rates are high

For asymptomatic patients, clinical practice is based on the results of two trials, the Asymptomatic Carotid Atherosclerosis Study (ACAS) and the Asymptomatic Carotid Atherosclerosis Surgery Trial (ACST) which concluded:
- in patients with >60% stenosis, the risk of ipsilateral stroke over 5 years is reduced with surgery and medical treatment compared with medical treatment alone (5% vs. 11%)
- risk of stroke within 30 days of surgery was 2.3% compared with 0.4% in the medical group alone in the same time period
- risk of stroke was reduced with immediate surgery compared with delayed surgery (3.8% vs. 11%)

What are the surgical treatment options?

- Carotid angioplasty and stenting: encouraging results but no published randomised trials
- Carotid endarterectomy: can be performed under LA or GA. Intraoperatively, it is imperative to prevent any fluctuations in BP and cerebral oxygenation. A shunt is used to maintain blood flow to the brain during clamping of the carotid artery

How can cerebral function be monitored in a patient undergoing carotid endarterectomy?

- Use of local anaesthetic with the patient awake
- Transcranial doppler
- Electroencephalogram (EEG)
- Transcranial PO_2 monitoring
- Stump pressure measurement

■ Clinical Governance

What do you understand by the term clinical governance?

Clinical governance is a framework through which NHS organisations are accountable for continuously improving the quality of care, and ensures that there is accountability within NHS Trusts and that there is a comprehensive programme of quality improvement systems. This is achieved through six facets listed below.

- Clinical effectiveness: is intervention efficient and safe?; guidance from National Service Framework (NSF), National Institute for Clinical Governance (NICE) and Commission for Healthcare Audit and Inspection (CHAI)
- Clinical audit: a process by which current practice is compared against a gold standard, any deficiencies identified and amended and a re-audit performed to ensure the changes have taken place thus 'closing the audit loop'. Audits can be of three types:
  - structure audit: type of resources
  - process: what is done to patients
  - outcome: results of clinical intervention
- Risk management: a risk is anything that may be hazardous to the patient, practitioner or to the NHS organisation. Personally we should ensure that guidelines and protocols are in place and followed. Dangerous situations should be reported either to departmental clinical governance committee or via critical incidence reports. Risk management involves four steps:
  1. identify the risk
  2. assess the frequency and severity of risk

3. reduce or eliminate the risk
4. cost the risk
- Education and Training: continuing personal development (CPD)
- Development and research
- Openness to the public

Is clinical audit like research?

Clinical audit and research are closely related but distinct disciplines. Research is about creating new knowledge about whether treatments work or whether one treatment works better than another. Clinical audit is about making sure that this knowledge is being used to best effect. Clinical audit and research can both look at the outcomes of treatment, but for different reasons. Research might observe outcomes to find out if a treatment works whereas clinical audit might monitor outcomes to ensure that best practice is producing the results we know (from research) that it should. The process of conducting clinical audit may identify areas where new research is needed.

■ Colitis

List the common causes of colitis
- Infection
- Ischaemia
- Radiation
- Inflammatory bowel disease
  - Crohn's disease
  - Ulcerative colitis
- Drugs
  - broad spectrum antibiotics (especially clindamycin)

What are the clinical features of inflammatory bowel disease?
Crohn's disease and ulcerative colitis are both characterised by:
- rectal bleeding
- mucus discharge
- abdominal pain (often relieved with defecation)
- altered bowel habit (usually diarrhoea)
- anaemia
- anorexia
- weight loss

List the extra-intestinal manifestations of inflammatory bowel disease
- Eyes
  - episcleritis
  - uveitis
  - conjunctivitis
- Joints

- monoarticular arthritis (usually affects knees and ankles)
- ankolysing spondylitis
- sacroilitis
- Skin
  - erythema nodosum
  - pyoderma gangrenosum
- Hepatobiliary
  - sclerosing cholangitis
  - chronic active hepatitis
  - hepatic cirrhosis
  - cholangiocarcinoma
- Calculi
  - renal
  - gall bladder

What are the histological differences between Crohn's disease and ulcerative colitis?

Crohn's disease	Ulcerative colitis
Microscopic	
• Transmural inflammation	• Mucosal inflammation
• Non-caseating granulomata	• No granulomata but goblet cell depletion and crypt abscesses
Macroscopic	
• Affects any part of the G.I. tract	• Affects the colon and rectum only
• Rectum is spared in 50%	• Always involves the rectum
• Terminal ileum involved in 30%	• Terminal ileum involved in 10%
• Discontinuous involvement ('skip lesions')	• Continuous involvement
• Deep mucosal ulcers and fissures ('cobblestone appearance')	• No fissuring

(*cont.*)

Crohn's disease	Ulcerative colitis

• Fistula formation in 15%–30%
  • enterocutaneous
  • enterovesical
  • enterovaginal
  • 'high-low' gastro-intestinal
	• Fistulae rare

• Perianal lesions in 75%
  • fistula and abscess
  • fissure
  • ulceration
  • skin tags
  • stenosis of anorectal junction
	• Perianal lesions in 20%

• 4–20× greater risk of small and large bowel malignancy than that of the general population.	• 10%–20% chance of developing colorectal carcinoma within 20 years of diagnosis

What are the medical treatment options in inflammatory bowel disease?

- 5-Aminosalicylic acid (5-ASA), e.g. Sulfasalazine, Mesalazine
  - blocks the production of prostaglandins and leukotrienes
  - used in mild or moderate cases of Crohn's disease or UC
- Corticosteroids
  - used to treat acute exacerbations and the dose tailed off as symptoms improve
  - proctosigmoiditis can be treated locally with steroid enemas and suppositories
- Immunosuppressive agents
  - Azathioprine is used in some patients to maintain a steroid-induced remission
  - Cyclosporin is used in the treatment of refractory UC

- Metronidazole
  - useful in severe perianal Crohn's disease

What are the indications for surgery in inflammatory bowel disease?
- Emergency
  - intestinal perforation
  - intestinal obstruction
  - haemorrhage
  - acute severe colitis unresponsive to medical therapy
  - toxic colonic dilatation
- Elective
  - chronic symptoms unresponsive to medical therapy
  - failure to thrive in children
  - intra-abdominal abscess/fistula (Crohn's disease)
  - persistent perianal disease (Crohn's disease)
  - carcinoma or high grade dysplasia (ulcerative colitis)

What are the principles of surgery in inflammatory bowel disease?
Due to the differences in the disease pattern between Crohn's disease and ulcerative colitis (UC), the principles of surgery are not the same. In Crohn's disease, surgical resection should be confined to the segment of symptomatic disease only whilst minimising the removal of normal gut because: relapse and recurrence are common and can affect the entire length of the G.I. tract and therefore cannot be 'cured' by surgery; and patients have a lifetime of the disease and therefore it is imperative to leave as much functioning bowel as possible. In contrast, radical surgery is often performed in UC because the disease is restricted to the large bowel and rectum and is always continuous and therefore removal of the affected segment may well cure the patient. Furthermore,

patients with chronic UC have an increased risk of developing colorectal carcinoma, which can be prevented by panproctocolectomy.

What are the surgical options in inflammatory bowel disease?

Emergency surgery:
- Sub-total colectomy with ileostomy and mucous fistula
  - quick surgical procedure with minimal surgical trauma, which reduces morbidity especially in sick patients
  - leaves an intact rectum and anal sphincter for future restorative surgery

Elective surgery:
- Panproctocolectomy with ileostomy
  - curative surgery for UC, which also eliminates the risk of future malignancy
  - leaves the patient with a permanent ileostomy so may not be popular with younger patients
- Sphincter-preserving proctocolectomy with ileal pouch
  - popular in younger patients with UC
  - complete continence achieved in 90% with mean stool frequency of 4–6/day
- Total colectomy with ileorectal anastomosis
  - used to avoid an ileostomy in UC and Crohn's disease whilst maintaining continence
  - optimal results achieved when the rectum is either not affected or only minimally affected
  - anastomosis should be avoided if there is an abscess cavity present close to the site of anastomosis, if serum albumin is low or if there is severe malnutrition

■ Colorectal Cancer

What are the risk factors for the development of colorectal cancer?

Approximately 75% of colorectal cancers are sporadic and develop in people with no known risk factors. The remaining are associated with risk factors listed below.

- Genetic factors (15%–20%):
  - hereditary non-polyposis colorectal cancer (HNPCC)
  - familial adenomatous polyposis (FAP)
- Inflammatory bowel disease (1%): incidence in ulcerative colitis is approximately 1% per year; incidence in patients with Crohn's disease is 4–20x greater than that of the general population
- Age: 80% of patients who develop colorectal cancer are >60 years of age
- Hereditary factors
  - family history: relative risk increases with the number of first-degree relatives affected and if the relative is <45 years at the time of diagnosis
  - personal history of colorectal cancer or polyps: 3% of patients with a successfully treated colon cancer will develop a further colorectal tumour within 10 years (metachronous tumour)
- Diet: a diet high in unsaturated animal fats, highly saturated vegetable oils and low fibre increases risk
- Alcohol: daily consumption increases risk by 2x
- Irradiation: pelvic irradiation increases risk of developing rectosigmoid carcinoma
- Previous cholecystectomy: not proven conclusively

What is the role of screening in colorectal cancers?

Colorectal cancer meets the WHO criteria for screening. Screening can be divided into two groups.

- Screening patients with a high risk is well established and involves testing:
  - relatives of those with FAP and HNPCC: examining for APC and MMR gene mutations respectively; regular colonoscopy for patients with HNPCC and those positive for APC gene mutation
  - those with ulcerative colitis for >10 yrs: yearly colonoscopy and serial biopsy for dysplasia
- Screening for the remaining sporadic cases: a national Bowel Cancer Screening Programme will be phased in from 2006 and rolled out over a 3-year period. Men and women aged 60–69 will be invited to take part in screening every 2 years. The screening test used will be faecal occult blood testing (FOBT) which is cheap, safe and performed in the privacy of patient's home; however it has limited sensitivity because not all polyps/cancers bleed and specificity is low because dietary factors (red meat, raw vegetables and fruit) can give false-positive results, which may result in unnecessary colonoscopy

Briefly describe the pathophysiology of carcinoma formation in people with polyps

In normal mucosa, the surface epithelium regenerates every 6–7 days. Crypt cells migrate from the base to the surface, where they undergo differentiation, maturation, and ultimately apoptosis. In adenomas (particularly villous type), a sequence of genetic mutations changes this process, starting with APC gene, permitting unhindered cellular replication at the crypt surface. Mutations of the tumour suppressor genes K-*ras* and *p53* prevent the cells being forced into apoptosis and allow replication of damaged cells. Through such mutations, changes in epithelium take place from normality, through dysplasia to invasion.

What is the distribution of carcinoma within the large bowel?

- Rectum (50%)
- Sigmoid (25%)
- Transverse and descending colon (12.5%)
- Caecum and ascending colon (12.5%): increase incidence in patients with FAP and HNPCC

What is the clinical presentation of colorectal carcinoma?

- Right-sided lesions: iron deficiency anaemia (secondary to chronic GI blood loss), weight loss, right iliac fossa mass
- Left-sided lesions: lower abdominal pain, altered bowel habit, rectal bleeding, tenesmus or rectal pain (rectal cancer)
- Emergency presentation: obstruction or perforation

Which investigations may be useful in the diagnosis and management of colorectal cancer?

- Bloods
  - FBC and U and Es
  - LFTs: often normal even with liver metastases
  - carcinoembryonic antigen (CEA): CEA >100 ng/ml usually indicates metastatic disease
- Flexible sigmoidoscopy: can detect polyps or cancers up to 60 cm from the anus
- Colonoscopy:
  - allows direct visualisation of the lesion
  - provides an estimation of the size of lesion and degree of obstruction

- allows biopsies to be taken
- gives an accurate measurement of the distance of the lesion from the dentate line, which is crucial in deciding the type of surgery to be offered
- Endorectal ultrasound (ERUS): allows assessment of depth of invasion of rectal cancer, presence of local recurrence when used after surgery and lymph node involvement
- CXR: to assess for pulmonary metastases and allows staging of tumour
- Double-contrast barium enemas: can miss lesions around the ileocaecal valve, in the distal rectum or in patients with severe diverticulosis
- CT:
  - determines presence or absence of metastases
  - helps determine if patients require pre-operative chemo-radiation therapy
  - helpful in follow-up of patients with resected cancers to assess for recurrence
  - can document response to chemotherapy
- MRI: the most sensitive test for determining the presence of liver metastases and often used if liver resection is considered
- Positron emission tomography (PET): differentiates between recurrent tumour and scar tissue

What are the principles of surgery for colorectal cancer?

Pre-operative:
- optimise fitness for anaesthesia
- establish location and extent of local disease including presence of any synchronous lesions
- determine tumour stage
- radiotherapy can reduce local recurrence, increases time to recurrence and improves 5-year survival rate

- bowel preparation: using polyethylene glycol or sodium picosulphate; in emergency cases, on table lavage may be performed
- prophylactic antibiotics: usually cephalosporin and metronidazole

Operative:

- in curable cases a wide resection is essential: 5 cm proximal and 2 cm distal clearance for colonic lesions and 2 cm distal clearance for rectal lesions (1 cm adequate if mesorectum resected)
- radial margin should be histologically free of tumour if possible
- lymph node resection should be performed to the origin of the feeding vessel
- fixity to, or invasion of, contiguous organs (bladder, uterus, stomach) should be treated with *en bloc* resection
- surgical options in non-obstructed cases are dependent on location of tumour:
  - caecum/ascending colon, hepatic flexure: right hemicolectomy
  - transverse colon: extended right hemicolectomy
  - splenic flexure/ descending colon: left hemicolectomy
  - sigmoid colon: left hemicolectomy or high anterior resection
  - high rectum: anterior resection
  - low rectum: abdomino-perineal resection and end-ileostomy
- consider defunctioning loop ileostomy if anastomosis <12 cm from anal margin
- for high rectal cancers, risk of local recurrence reduced by performing total mesorectal excision (TME)
- consider liver resection if disease confined to a single lobe without involvement of the major vessels and no evidence of extrahepatic disease

- in obstructed emergency cases, decompression should be followed by elective surgery if necessary
- in incurable cases, relieve present or potential obstruction

Post-operative:
- hydration with iv fluids until normal oral intake has resumed
- continue with prophylactic antibiotics (at least three post-operative doses)
- colostomy care
- thromboembolic prophylaxis

What are the specific complications of surgery?
- Anastomotic leak: occurs 7–10 d post-surgery; risk higher in lower anastomoses
- Anastomotic stricture
- Intestinal obstruction
- Injury to the urinary tract
- Sexual dysfunction:
  - impotence: seen after AP and anterior resection (injury to nervi erigentes)
  - failure of ejaculation: damage to presacral nerves
  - dyspareunia in women due to fibrosis around the vagina
- Phantom rectum: sensation of an uncomfortable rectum after AP resection
- Colostomy complications

How are colorectal tumours classified?
- Adenocarcinoma (98%): polypoid, ulcerating, annular
- Rare types (2%): carcinoid, lymphoma, leiomyosarcoma

How are colorectal tumours staged?
Dukes' ABC system: devised for rectal carcinomas but is now used for rectal and colonic carcinomas. The classification has been modified to include two 'B' and 'C' categories as well as a 'D' category to represent distant metastases.

Stage	Definition	Five-year survival (%)
A	spread to sub-mucosa but not muscle	90
B	spread to muscle but node negative	70
C	lymph node metastases present	40

What is the role of adjuvant therapy post-operatively?

- Chemotherapy: currently being investigated in the QUASAR (Quick and Simple and Reliable) trial. Results so far show:
  - improves survival in Duke's C tumours
  - some benefit in Duke's B tumours in patients with adverse prognostic indicators
  - not required in Duke's A tumours, which already have a good prognosis
  - 5FU and folinic acid is effective as adjuvant therapy
- Radiotherapy: usually only offered to patients with high risk of recurrence

Compartment Syndrome I: Extremities

Define compartment syndrome

It is elevation of interstitial pressure in a closed myofascial compartment that results in microvascular compromise and organ dysfunction.

Outline the pathophysiology resulting in compartment syndrome

Intra-compartmental structures cannot withstand infinite pressure. As intra-compartmental pressure (ICP) increases, venous pressure rises and eventually causes capillaries to collapse. Blood flow through the capillaries stops and in the absence of flow, oxygen delivery stops. Hypoxic injury causes cells to release vasoactive substances (e.g. histamine, serotonin), which increase endothelial permeability. Capillaries allow continued fluid loss, which increases tissue pressure and aggravates the ischaemic insult. A vicious cycle of rising pressures is thus created. Arterial inflow is reduced when ICP exceeds systolic blood pressure.

What is the aetiology of compartment syndrome?

Decreased compartment size secondary to:
- Prolonged limb compression:
  - tight plaster casts or dressings
  - tourniquets
- Closure of fascial defects
- Burns
- Military antishock trousers (MAST)

Increased compartmental contents secondary to:

- Bleeding:
  - vascular injury
  - bleeding disorders
  - anticoagulation therapy
- Reduced capillary permeability:
  - trauma (fractures, soft tissue injury, crush injury)
  - intensive muscle use (e.g. tetany, vigorous exercise, seizures)
  - intra-arterial drug injection
  - post-ischaemic swelling
- Increased capillary pressure:
  - venous obstruction
  - muscle hypertrophy
  - nephrotic syndrome
  - infiltration of infusions

Does compartment syndrome only occur in closed fractures?

No. It is more common in comminuted and type 3 open fractures.

What are the symptoms and signs?

- Pain out of proportion to the injury (most important symptom)
- Pain on stretching the involved compartment (most reliable sign)
- Muscle tenderness
- Pallor of the extremity
- Paralysis
- Paraesthesia in the distribution of nerves passing through the compartment (early loss of vibratory sensation)
- Peripheral pulses may still be present

How is it diagnosed?

- Clinical diagnosis
- Measurement of intra-compartmental pressure (ICP). The critical pressure for diagnosing compartment pressure remains unclear but surgical intervention is indicated if:
  - absolute ICP > 30 mmHg
  - difference between diastolic pressure and ICP < 30 mmHg
  - difference between mean arterial pressure and ICP < 40 mmHg

What is the treatment?

- Remove any constricting casts or dressings that may cause limb compression
- If there is no improvement urgent fasciotomy is required. The skin and deep fascia along the whole length of the compartment must be divided and the wound left open

Describe chronic (exertional) compartment syndrome

- Most often occurs in the anterior or lateral lower tibial compartments
- Symptoms are exercise related, which recover quickly after resting from the inciting activity
- Diagnosis is difficult, but compartment pressures should be checked. Thallium stress testing can augment pressure monitoring
- Treatment is conservative with rest from the aggravating activity but symptoms return on re-commencing activities. Fasciotomy may be indicated if conservative treatment fails. Deep posterior compartment does not respond as quickly or as well to fasciotomy as the anterior compartment

Compartment Syndrome II: Abdominal

What are the causes of abdominal compartment syndrome (ACS)?

- Primary: intra-abdominal pathology directly causes the compartment syndrome
  - penetrating trauma
  - gastrointestinal haemorrhage
  - pancreatitis
  - pelvic fracture
  - rupture of abdominal aortic aneurysm
  - perforated peptic ulcer
- Secondary: injuries outside the abdomen cause fluid accumulation
  - sepsis
  - burns
  - penetrating or blunt trauma without identifiable injury
  - postoperative
- Chronic:
  - advanced liver cirrhosis
  - ascites
  - peritoneal dialysis
  - morbid obesity
  - Meigs syndrome

Describe the pathophysiology of ACS?

Although the abdominal cavity is more distensible than an extremity, it can reach an endpoint at which the pressure rises dramatically. With rising pressures, many organ systems are affected, e.g.

- pressure over the splanchnic circulation causes gut ischaemia
- renal vascular insufficiency causes oliguria
- raised intra-thoracic and airway pressures cause pulmonary dysfunction
- compression of the inferior vena cava reduces venous return and cardiac output
- intra-cranial pressure rises

What are the symptoms and signs of ACS?
- Abdominal pain
- Distended abdomen: Cullen or Grey–Turner signs
- Wheezing; difficulty in breathing; increased respiratory rate
- Decreased urinary frequency
- Syncope
- Malena
- Nausea and vomiting

How is ACS diagnosed?
- High index of clinical suspicion
- Abdominal CT scan: shows abdominal distention with an increased ratio of anteroposterior-to-transverse abdominal diameter, collapse of the vena cava, bowel wall thickening with enhancement or bilateral inguinal herniation
- Intra-abdominal pressure (IAP) estimation by measuring intra-luminal bladder pressure. Normal values for IAP are between 0 and 6 mmHg. Pressures > 22–25 mmHg indicate the presence or imminent development of ACS

What are the treatment options?
- Prevention: focused on early treatment of intra-abdominal hypertension by proactive pressure measurement and monitoring
- Remove any constricting garments

- Drugs to reduce intra-abdominal pressure, e.g. diuretics
- Percutaneous fluid drainage: particularly useful in patients with chronic ACS secondary to ascites and in burns patients
- Laparoscopic decompression: mainly used for blunt abdominal trauma
- Open surgical decompression

What is the mortality rate with ACS?

Approximately 50%.

■ Consent

What types of consent are there?
- Express consent:
  - required in all procedures with possible complications, e.g. surgery, OGD
  - can be written or oral
- Implied consent:
  - consent is assumed when the patient complies with a particular action, e.g. physical examination

What are the principles of good consent?
- It should take place in a suitable environment
- The use of simple language
- The doctor should explain the procedure, its benefits and risks, the prognosis and any alternative treatments with their associated risks and benefits
- Patients should understand the information, retain it and be able to weigh up the benefits and risks of the procedure

When is consent required?
- In all procedures requiring a general anaesthetic
- In procedures under local anaesthetic or sedation with possible complications

Why is consent required?
- Moral obligation
- Legal obligation – failure to obtain informed consent can result in charges of battery or negligence

Who can obtain consent?

Only those who are adequately trained and qualified and have sufficient knowledge of the proposed treatment and its risks.

What is Bolam's law?

Amount of information is adequate if it accords with accepted medical practice.

What is the difference between battery and negligence?

Battery is a violation of civil law which forbids intentionally touching another person without consent (it does not have to result in physical harm).

Negligence is a lack of professional duty on the doctor's part to properly advise the patient on the procedure and its potential risks.

What are the principles of consent in children?

The legal age of consent is 16. For children below this age, a parent or legal guardian must provide consent on their behalf. A parent or legal guardian's wishes can be over-ridden by the doctor if it is thought to act in the child's best interests, although it is advisable to obtain a court order to do so.

Children under the age of 16 can provide consent if they are deemed competent (Gillick's principle). If a competent child refuses treatment, the parent or legal guardian can authorise treatment that is deemed to be in the child's best interests.

What are the principles of consent in unconscious and psychiatric patients?

In an unconscious patient, surgery can be performed without express consent if it is deemed to be in the best interest of the patient. Similarly, surgical treatment can be provided in psychiatric patients who are unable to provide informed consent because of their illness or if the surgery is necessary to protect their life or to avoid permanent disability.

In both these situations, although the patient's family are not legally able to provide consent on the patient's behalf, it is good surgical practice to obtain their approval.

Corticosteroid Therapy and Surgery

List the common conditions for which a patient might be taking corticosteroids
- Chronic obstructive pulmonary disease
- Inflammatory bowel disease
- Rheumatoid arthritis
- Malignancy
- Recipients of transplanted organs

What are the equivalent anti-inflammatory doses of hydrocortisone, dexamethasone and triamcinalone for 10 mg prednisolone?
- Hydrocortisone, 40 mg
- Dexamethasone, 12 mg
- Triamcinalone, 8 mg

What effect does surgery have on corticosteroid production?
In healthy patients, surgery causes a sharp increase ($2-3\times$) in cortisol output due to the stimulation of the hypothalamic–pituitary–adrenal axis and via cytokine-induced production. Patients on long-term corticosteroids may not be able to mount such a response and may suffer an Addisonian crisis.

What are the effects of corticosteroid deficiency?
- Hypotension
- Bradycardia
- Low systemic vascular resistance

- Cardiac failure
- Hypoglycaemia
- Confusion
- Coma

What are the main indications for perioperative corticosteroid cover?
- Patients on systemic steroid therapy of >7.5 mg for >1 week before surgery
- Patients who have had a course of steroids for >1 month in the preceding year
- Patients undergoing pituitary or adrenal surgery
- Patients with established pituitary–adrenal insufficiency
- Septic shock
- Previous use of etomidate

What is the regimen for peri-operative and post-operative corticosteroid cover?

Type of surgery	Pre-operative hydrocortisone dose	Post-operative hydrocortisone dose
Minor	25–50 mg iv/im	
Intermediate	50–75 mg iv/im	50–75 mg iv/im for 24 h
Major	100 mg iv	100 mg iv qds for 24 h
		100 mg iv bd for next 24 h
		50 mg iv bd until stopped

When should hydrocortisone be stopped?
When patients are able to resume their normal oral therapy or when they have recovered from the stress period, in patients not on regular corticosteroid therapy.

What are the effects of high dose peri-operative corticosteroid treatment?

- Delayed wound healing
- Increased risk of infection
- Metabolic effects (hypernatraemia, hypokalaemia, metabolic alkalosis)
- Addisonian crisis

■ Day Surgery

Currently what proportion of elective surgery is performed as day cases?
50%. This is likely to increase further in the future.

What are the benefits of day surgery?
- Less disruption to the patient
- Increased availability of in-patient beds
- Less cost
- Reduction in hospital-acquired infections
- Reduction of in-patient waiting lists

Which operations are suitable for day cases?
Procedures which:
- are of short duration (<1 h)
- have low complication rates
- have minimal blood loss
- do not require post-operative intravenous fluids
- do not require prolonged post-operative monitoring
- do not require strong opioid base analgesia post-operatively

Which patients are suitable for day surgery?
- ASA grades I or II
- Age <70
- BMI <35
- Patients with well-controlled mild systemic disease (e.g. asthma, hypertension)
- Those who live in close proximity to the hospital

When should patients be discharged from day case unit?

Patients should only be discharged when they:

- are comfortable
- have a GCS of 15
- have stable vital signs
- are tolerating fluids
- are able to pass urine
- are able to stand erect with their eyes shut
- have minimal nausea and vomiting
- are able to dress themselves

What instructions should be given to patients on discharge?

- They must not drive or operate machinery for at least 24 h post-surgery
- They must be accompanied home
- They must have a responsible adult to look after them overnight
- They should seek immediate medical attention if there are any problems

■ Diabetes and Surgery

What are the systemic complications of diabetes mellitus?
- Cardiovascular:
  - hypertension
  - ischaemic heart disease
  - peripheral vascular disease
  - cardiomyopathy
- Respiratory:
  - reduced FEV_1 : FVC ratio
- Renal impairment:
  - nephropathy: many patients end up with end-stage renal failure
- Autonomic neuropathy
- Metabolic disturbances:
  - hypoglycaemia, hyperglycaemia and ketoacidosis
- Impaired polymorphonuclear leukocyte function
- Retinopathy

What are the particular risks of anaesthesia in diabetic patients?
- General anaesthesia masks the signs of hypoglycaemia and reduces the neuro-endocrine response to hypoglycaemia
- Inhalational anaesthetic agents can cause hyperglycaemia which if untreated can cause ketoacidosis and coma
- The presence of cardiovascular diseases will increase the incidence of intra-operative myocardial infarction and CVA in anaesthetised patients

- Autonomic neuropathy can cause unexpected tachycardia, hypotension and even cardiac arrest in anaesthetised patients
- Autonomic neuropathy can cause delayed gastric emptying and increase the risk of aspiration
- Intubation or other hypertensive manoeuvres can cause vitreous haemorrhage in patients with retinopathy

What are the particular risks of surgery in diabetic patients?

Diabetic patients have an increased incidence of wound, respiratory and urinary tract infections post-operatively

How should diabetic patients be managed in the peri-operative period?

- Good pre-operative glycaemic control is essential and is directly associated with reduced post-operative complications. HbA1c of <8.0% indicates adequate glycaemic control over the last 8 weeks
- Optimise any associated medical conditions
- Ensure the patient is listed first on the operating list

How should these patients be managed prior to surgery?

- In diet-controlled patients, the patient should be fasted 6 h before surgery and capillary glucose monitored four times a day. They must not receive intravenous dextrose fluid replacement
- In oral hypoglycaemic controlled patients undergoing minor surgery, the morning dose of their tablets should be omitted. Capillary glucose is monitored 4-hourly and oral hypoglycaemic agents commenced only once the patient is eating and drinking normally

If these patients are undergoing major surgery or surgery in which there are restrictions to eating in the post-operative period then as well as omitting their hypoglycaemic agents on the morning of the surgery, a glucose insulin infusion (sliding scale) should be commenced 2 hours before surgery.

For afternoon theatre lists, oral hypoglycaemic agents (except long-acting agents such as sulphonylureas) can be taken on the morning of surgery and a glucose insulin infusion (sliding scale) commenced 2 hours before surgery

- In insulin-controlled patients undergoing minor surgery, the morning insulin dose is omitted until after the procedure. For those on the afternoon theatre list, an early breakfast and half the usual morning dose of insulin should be given. Lunchtime insulin is omitted until after the procedure.

If these patients are undergoing major surgery or surgery in which there are restrictions to eating in the post-operative period, then no insulin should be given on the morning of surgery and a glucose insulin infusion commenced 2 hours before surgery.

For afternoon theatre lists, half the usual morning dose of insulin should be given before breakfast and glucose insulin infusion commenced 2 hours before surgery.

How should they be monitored in the intra-operative and post-operative periods?

Intra-operatively, hypoglycaemia should be avoided and capillary glucose monitored regularly (about every 2 h) with an aim to achieve plasma glucose between 5–7 mmol/l. Post-operatively, capillary glucose should be measured pre-meal and at bedtime after minor surgery and 4-hourly after major surgery.

Post-operatively, insulin requirements are often increased and patients may require higher dosage than their usual dose. Glycaemic control can be disturbed for some time after discharge and patients should be given appropriate advice by the hospital diabetic unit regarding managing their glucose levels.

■ Diathermy

How does diathermy work?

It works by passage of high frequency alternating current through body tissues to produce heat. Safe passage of currents up to 500 mA at frequencies between 400 kHz to 10 MHz can be introduced. Neuromuscular activation does not occur at frequencies above 10 kHz. In cutting mode, the high temperature causes cellular water to explode. In coagulation mode, tissue damage occurs by fulguration. In 'touching' mode, tissue dehydration and protein denaturation occurs.

What temperature is produced by cutting surgical diathermy?

Up to 1000 °C!

What are the different diathermy settings?

- Cutting mode: continuous output of low frequency currents in a sinus wave form
- Coagulation mode: pulsed output of high frequency currents at short intervals in a square wave form
- Blend mode: continuous sine wave current with superimposed bursts of higher intensity

How does bipolar diathermy work?

A low power unit (50 W) generates low frequencies. The current passes between the two limbs of diathermy forceps only. A patient plate electrode (PPE) is not needed.

How does monopolar diathermy work?

A high power unit (400 W) generates high frequencies. The current passes from the active electrode (high current density), held by the surgeon, through the patient's body and returns to the generator (low current density) via the patient plate electrode.

Where should the patient plate electrode be placed?

- On dry shaved skin
- On at least 70 cm^2 contact surface area
- Away from bony prominences and scar tissues
- Away from metallic implants

What are the advantages of bipolar diathermy over monopolar diathermy?

Bipolar diathermy is safer than monopolar and should be used for surgery on end arteries. However, monopolar diathermy has to be used for cutting and touching instruments. In patients with pacemakers, bipolar diathermy should be used. If monopolar diathermy has to be used, ensure PPE is away from the heart and use short bursts (<2 s) at long intervals.

What are the complications of using diathermy?

- Electrocution
- Burns (especially if alcohol-based skin preparation used)
- Can interfere with pacemaker function
- Channelling – if used on viscus with narrow pedicle (e.g. penis)
- Explosion (especially in obstructed hollow viscera)

What are the specific complications of using diathermy during laparoscopic surgery?

- Direct coupling: occurs if diathermy is in contact with a second metallic instrument and the electric current flows through it causing a burn if the current cannot dissipate through a large surface area

- Capacitance coupling: capacitance occurs when a non-conductor of electricity separates two conductors. This typically occurs between an insulted instrument and a metal cannula. An electrostatic current field is created and it can induce current in the metal cannula. Plastic cannula does not eliminate this problem completely as the patient's body can act as a conductor. The worst situation occurs when a metal trocar is used in a plastic cannula and therefore the use of plastic-metal hybrid instruments should be avoided
- Retained heat: in tips of diathermy forceps

■ Drains

What materials are drains made of?
- Latex-based materials
- PVC
- Silastic
- Polyurethane

What are the indications for insertion of a drain?
- To drain an established collection, e.g. pus, blood or lymphatic fluid
- To remove anticipated collections after surgery, e.g. after AP resection
- As prophylaxis to abolish dead space

Classify drains
- Active or passive
- Open or closed

How can active closed drains be further classified?
- Re-usable: a high pressure suction system (typically 500 mmHg) connected to a reservoir (bottle) of varying capacity. Bottles can be autoclaved for re-use
- Disposable: a low pressure suction system (typically 100 mmHg) connected to a compressible bottle via a non-return valve which prevents reflux. System can be re-charged by emptying the bottle, compressing and re-connecting the drainage tube. Since these drainage systems are never completely empty, they are prone to colonisation by organisms

How do active open drains work?

They contain an air inlet lumen which prevents blockage by soft tissues. Although more efficient than closed suction drains, they have the disadvantage of requiring a non-portable suction system and may permit entry of bacteria (this can be reduced by using filters).

Describe passive drains

- Closed system: drain into bags by low pressure suction working on siphon principle
- Open system: drain by capillary action or gravity into dressings or stoma bags therefore their efficiency is influenced by the position of patient, volume and site of collection

How long should drains be used for?

Drains should be removed within 5 days of insertion unless the daily volume is large. If a track is necessary to provide long-term drainage, e.g. biliary t-tube, then rubber drains should be used as they stimulate tissue fibrosis.

What are the disadvantages of drains?

- Infection: higher incidence in open than closed drains; infection rates can be reduced by use of non-return valves
- Haemorrhage
- Pressure or suction necrosis leading to leakage of contents, e.g. following bowel anastomosis
- It can give an incorrect notion of bleeding when it is blocked
- They can be painful if they are in contact with sensitive areas

■ Dressings

What properties should a 'perfect' dressing possess?

There are no dressings on the market which encompass all the ideal properties listed below and therefore the dressing should be selected according to each individual case. A dressing should:

- promote healing of a wound
- maintain a moist wound environment
- protect the wound from contamination and trauma
- be comfortable and easy to change
- remove excess exudates, without saturating the dressing to its outer surface
- allow gaseous exchange
- be cosmetically acceptable
- be inexpensive
- reduce wound odour

How do vacuum-assisted dressings work?

A piece of foam with an open-cell structure is introduced into the wound and a wound drain with lateral perforations laid on top of it. The entire area is covered with an occlusive adhesive membrane. The foam dressing is connected to a vacuum source which provides a uniform negative pressure (50–125 mmHg) over the wound bed.

The negative pressure allows removal of interstitial fluid, reducing localised oedema and enhancing blood flow. This in turn reduces tissue bacterial levels. Additionally, mechanical deformation of cells is thought to result in protein and matrix molecule synthesis, which increases the rate of cell proliferation.

What are the indications and contraindications for the use of vacuum-assisted dressings?

Indications are wounds which are:
- large
- deep and produce excessive exudates

Contra-indications include:
- local malignancy
- presence of fistulas
- wounds with exposed organs

What are the indications for the use of biological dressings?

The larvae of the common greenbottle fly secrete enzymes which breakdown necrotic tissues and can be used in treating sloughing or necrotic wounds.

List some commonly used dressings with their advantages and disadvantages

Dressing type	Made from	Use	Advantages	Disadvantages
Alginates (Sorbasan, Kaltostat)	Sodium or calcium alginate	Exudating wounds, bleeding wounds	Can have haemostatic properties; absorb exudates; easy removal	Require frequent changing; cannot be used on dry wounds
Tulle (Jelonet)	Cotton/ viscose gauze impregnated with paraffin	Superficial clean wounds, burns, ulcers, skin grafts, traumatic wounds	Easy to remove; prevents moisture absorption from wound	Require frequent changing; skin sensitisation
Low adherence (Mepore)	Variety of materials, e.g. viscose, polyester	Superficial wounds, lightly exudating wounds	Cheap; durable; minimal dressing adherence	Maceration of surrounding tissues

Dressing type	Made from	Use	Advantages	Disadvantages
Hydrocolloids (Granuflex)	Hydrocolloid matrix of gelatine, pectin and cellulose	Leg ulcers, pressure sores, granulating wounds, burns	Durable; cheap; waterproof; absorb exudates; promotes granulation tissue formation	Not suitable for cavities; can cause an odour; can be difficult to remove
Hydrofibres (Aquacel)	Polyurethane	Contributes to wound debridement	Highly absorbent; comfortable	Expensive
Hydrogels (Aquaform)	Starch polymers with high water content	Dry necrotic and sloughing wounds	Absorbent; comfortable; conform to wound shape; permit water to pass into wound	Expensive; frequent changing, difficult to retain on wound
Foam (Allevyn)	Polyurethane	Outer dressing with other products	Permeable to water/gases; thermal insulation; protection; absorbs exudates and fluids from wound	Expensive; can only be used on flat surfaces
Films (Opsite)	Polyurethane	Superficial wounds, lightly exudating, epithelialising wounds	Comfortable; waterproof; allows gaseous exchange	Fluid collection can cause maceration; only suitable for flat surfaces

(*cont.*)

Dressing type	Made from	Use	Advantages	Disadvantages
Antimicrobial (Inadine)	Povidine-iodine impregnated	Infected wounds	Antibacterial	Sensitivity to product
Odour reducing (Actisorb)	Charcoal	Fungating or gangrenous wounds	Reduces wound odour	Expensive; not suitable for all wound types

Drugs in the Perioperative Period

Why is it important to elicit the patient's drug history during pre-assessment?

- Drugs can interfere with general anaesthetic agents. For example, monoamine oxidase inhibitor (MAOI) antidepressants can cause cardiac crisis with general anaesthesia and must be stopped at least 2 weeks before surgery
- Drugs given in hospital can interfere with the patient's normal drugs. For example, women taking combined oral contraceptive should take other contraceptive measures if they receive broad spectrum antibiotics perioperatively, as alterations in the bowel flora can decrease their efficiency
- Drugs may need to be started in the perioperative period. For example,
  - peri-operative administration of beta-adrenoreceptor blockade can reduce the risk of intra- and post-operative cardiovascular complications
  - glucose-insulin infusions may need to be started in diabetic patients
- Drugs may need to be stopped in the perioperative period. For example,
  - oral anticoagulants should be stopped or its effects reversed depending on indication for surgery
  - aspirin may need to be stopped up to 7 days before surgery to minimise perioperative blood loss
  - oestrogen containing oral contraceptives should be stopped at least 4 weeks before surgery to reduce the risk of deep vein thrombosis

- lithium should be stopped 24 h prior to surgery
- hypoglycaemic agents need to be omitted on the day of surgery
- Drug doses may need to be changed in the perioperative period. For example, patients on corticosteroids are likely to require increased doses perioperatively
- Drug doses may need to be changed in the post-operative period. For example, insulin requirements are often increased following surgical trauma
- Discontinuation of chronic treatment can cause worsening of symptoms. For example, stopping the following drugs can cause serious consequences

• Anticonvulsants	• Convulsions, hypoxia
• Antihypertensives	• Hypertension, heart failure, stroke
• Antiarrhythmics	• Arrhythmias, embolism
• Antipsychotics	• Psychiatric disturbances
• Bronchodilators	• Exacerbation of symptoms, respiratory failure

■ Deep Venous Thrombosis (DVT)

Why is DVT prophylaxis important?

DVT occurs in about 50% of all patients undergoing major abdominal, pelvic or lower limb orthopaedic surgery, in the absence of thromboprophylaxis. About 20% of these patients will go on to develop pulmonary embolism (PE), of which up to 5% will be fatal. Prophylaxis reduces the incidence of post-operative DVT to less than 5%.

What are the main risk factors for DVT?

Factors which cause changes in:

- Blood flow: atheroma, immobility, prolonged surgery, plaster casts, obesity, trauma, compromised venous drainage
- Blood vessel wall: atheroma, vascular injury
- Blood constituents: smoking, oestrogen therapy, inherited deficiencies of protein C, protein S and antithrombin III, antiphospholipid antibody syndrome, pregnancy, obesity, malignancy

How can the risk of venous thromboembolism be stratified in surgical patients?

Risk	Type of surgery	Predisposing factors
Low (DVT <0.4%; PE <0.2%)	• Minor (<30 min) • Major (>30 min) • Any (in patients with minor trauma or illness with no thrombophilia but history of DVT/PE)	• No other risk factors • No other risk factors

(cont.)

(Cont.)

Risk	Type of surgery	Predisposing factors
Moderate (DVT 2–4%; PE 0.2–0.5%)	• Major (>30 min) • Minor (<30 min) • Any surgery in patients with major trauma or patients with major acute medical illness	• Age >40; one other risk factor • Previous DVT/PE or plaster cast immobilisation
High (DVT 10–20%; PE 1–5%)	• Major surgery for cancer • Critical leg ischaemia or lower limb amputation • Major surgery for pelvis, hip or leg or surgery for long bone fractures • Major pelvic or abdominal surgery	

What methods can be used to minimise the occurrence of DVT in surgical patients?

- Pre-operative:
  - cessation of smoking
  - cessation of oestrogens (OCP, HRT) at least 6 weeks before surgery
  - adequate hydration
  - graduated compression stockings
  - heel cushions to prevent pressure on calf veins
  - elevation of legs to promote venous drainage
  - pharmacological methods
- Operative:
  - appropriate patient positioning
  - adequate hydration
  - intermittent sequential pneumatic pressure devices
  - use of regional anaesthesia

- pharmacological methods
- Post-operative:
  - early mobilisation
  - graduated elastic compression stockings
  - intermittent sequential pneumatic pressure devices
  - heel cushions to prevent pressure on calf veins
  - elevation of legs to promote venous drainage
  - pharmacological methods

What are the pharmacological methods of DVT prophylaxis?

- Unfractionated heparin: inhibits thrombin. APTT needs to be monitored regularly. Side effects include: bleeding, thrombocytopenia, HITTS syndrome, osteoporosis
- Low molecular-weight heparin (LMWH): once daily administration only; fewer side effects and no requirement for APTT monitoring
- Warfarin: prevents synthesis of vitamin-K-dependent clotting factors in the liver. INR needs to be monitored regularly. It has numerous side effects and interacts with other medications
- Recombinant hirudin (desirudin): direct thrombin inhibitor. Has greater efficacy than LMWHs in thromboprophylaxis for hip replacement surgery
- Synthetic selective factor-Xa inhibitor (e.g. Fondaparinux): safe and effective but expensive. Its long half-life allows for once-daily dosing. No antidote in the event of overanticoagulation

What investigations may be useful in diagnosing a PE?

- Arterial blood gas: hypoxaemia with hypocapnia (but this is non-specific)

- ECG: usually normal but may show sinus tachycardia, right heart strain or $S_1Q_3T_3$ (rare)
- CXR: often normal but may show decreased vascular markings, raised hemidiaphragm, wedge shaped infarcts (large PEs only)
- Ventilation perfusion scan: shows areas of mismatch
- Pulmonary angiography (or CTPA): shows obstructed vessels or filling defects

■ Elderly and Surgery

What do you understand by the term 'functional reserve'?

Functional reserve is the difference between basal level of organ function at rest and the maximum level of organ function that can be achieved in response to increased demand, e.g. during exercise or in response to surgical stress. There is an age-dependent reduction in functional reserve, which is a major factor in the increased morbidity and mortality levels observed in the elderly.

What changes in organ function are found in the elderly?

- Cardiovascular:
  - ischaemic heart disease
  - hypertension
  - reduced cardiac output
  - atrial fibrillation (AF)
  - impaired physiological response to hypovolaemia due to reduced baroreceptor sensitivity and autonomic function
- Respiratory:
  - reduced pulmonary elasticity, lung and chest wall compliance, total lung capacity, FVC, FEV_1, vital capacity and inspiratory reserve volume (IRV)
  - increased residual volume
  - atelectasis, pulmonary embolism and chest infections are common, particularly following abdominal or thoracic surgery
- Renal:

- reduced cardiac output compromises renal and cerebral blood flow; autoregulation of blood flow to these organs is impaired in the elderly, and therefore both the kidneys and brain are prone to peri-operative ischaemia
  - reduced glomerular filtration
  - impaired tubular function
  - reduced clearance of renally excreted drugs
- Endocrine:
  - diabetes mellitus
- Nervous system:
  - pre- and post-operative confusion
  - cognitive impairment and dementia
- Pharmacology:
  - altered pharmacokinetics and pharmacodynamics resulting in increased free drug levels and increased sensitivity to many drugs
- Nutrition: malnutrition is common

What are the particular risks of anaesthesia in elderly patients?

- Autonomic dysfunction is common and may result in labile blood pressure and arrhythmias peri-operatively; baroreceptor reflex may be attenuated causing postural hypotension and a drop in blood pressure during anaesthesia
- Delayed gastric emptying can predispose the patient to aspiration
- Altered pharmacodynamics with increased sensitivity to many anaesthetic agents, e.g. isoflurane
- Osteoporosis and ligament laxity may make epidurals and spinals technically difficult
- Induction of anaesthesia: arm-brain circulation time is increased, and induction agent dose requirements reduced. An induction dose of propofol may result in hypotension

and require a vasopressor. Ketamine should be used with caution especially in those with cardiac disease as the tachycardia and hypertension that may result can increase myocardial oxygen consumption and precipitate ischaemia

- Elderly patients have a reduced basal metabolic rate (BMR) and are susceptible to heat loss as a result of impaired thermoregulation
- Hypotension is more commonly seen in elderly patients undergoing spinal/epidural anaesthesia due to impaired autonomic function

How should elderly patients be managed in the post-operative period?

- O_2 therapy especially following major surgery, in patients with cardiovascular or respiratory disease, surgery associated with blood loss, or when prescribing opioid analgesia
- Admission to HDU/ICU immediately postoperatively may improve long-term outcome
- Beware of prescribing NSAIDs: renal impairment and peptic ulceration are more common in older patients
- Meticulous fluid management: dehydration and fluid overload are a common cause of morbidity and mortality
- Regular review assessing for postoperative complications
- DVT prophylaxis: chemical agents, early mobilisation
- Rehabilitation using a multidisciplinary team

Empyema

Define empyema

Empyema is the collection of pus in a cavity bounded by mesothelium or epithelium. It is a form of abscess that most commonly affects the gall bladder or pleural cavity.

Describe empyema of the gall bladder

A gallstone which is lodged in Hartmanns's pouch of the gall bladder obstructs the flow of mucin. The glandular secretions accumulate and produce a mucocoele. If infection supervenes, it gives rise to an empyema of the gall bladder. The causative organisms are often enteric, usually *E. coli*, *Klebsiella*, *Streptococcus faecalis*, *Bacteroides* or *Clostridium perfringens*. Subsequent gangrene, perforation and peritonitis are likely if the gall bladder is not removed surgically or drained by cholecystostomy.

Describe empyema thoracis

A collection of purulent exudate or pus in the pleural cavity. Many patients are malnourished, cachectic or immunocompromised. The causes are:

- Local: infection of the pleura from adjacent lung (lung abscess, bronchiectasis or bronchial carcinoma) or from a penetrating injury
- Blood borne: *Streptococcus pneumoniae* or *milleri*, *Staphylococcus aureus*, *Klebsiella* and anaerobic organisms are the common pathogens. Infection may be derived via the diaphragm, classically with *Entamoeba histolytica*. Embolic infarcts from non-sterile talc which become infected are not uncommon in intravenous drug abusers.

The fungus *Aspergillus fumigatus* may cause empyema in the immunocompromised patient

- Most develop in the posterior and inferior parts of the pleural cavity
- Clinical features include dysponea, cough, pleuritic chest pain and pyrexia
- Diagnosis can be confirmed by CXR, USS or CT
- Management includes thoracentesis, intercostal drain insertion, thoracoscopic aided drainage or rib resection

■ Endocrine Disorders and Surgery

Why are patients with thyroid disorders at higher risk from surgical complications?

- They may have large goitres with retrosternal extension causing tracheal compression (can cause difficulties with airway maintenance and intubation) or recurrent laryngeal nerve palsy (can cause airway obstruction or stridor)
- They may have associated medical problems:
  - hypothyroid patients: macrocytic anaemia, bradycardia, cardiomegaly, ischaemic heart disease, pericardial effusion
  - hyperthyroid patients: tachycardia, atrial fibrillation, heart failure
- Patients should be rendered euthyroid prior to surgery otherwise they have high perioperative risks such as in:
  - hypothyroid patients: myocardial ischaemia, hypotension, hypoventilation, hypothermia, hypoglycaemia, hyponatraemia and coma
  - hyperthyroid patients: hypertension, cardiovascular instability and thyroid crisis (hyperthermia, arrhythmias, cardiorespiratory failure, coma) which can be fatal

Why are patients with parathyroid disorders at higher risk from surgical complications?

Hyperparathyroidism patients may have co-existing medical conditions such as:

- renal impairment secondary to hypercalcaemia (primary hyperparathyroidism) which will require appropriate

rehydration and treatment with diuretics. Severe cases may require dialysis prior to surgery
- chronic renal failure secondary to hypocalcaemia (Secondary and tertiary hyperparathyroidism)
- hypertension
- associated tumours, e.g. bronchial carcinomas which secrete PTH

Hypoparathyroid patients are at increased risk from the complications of untreated hypocalcaemia: poor cardiac output, stridor and convulsions

Why are patients with Cushing's syndrome high-risk surgical candidates?

- Anaesthetic difficulties due to proximal myopathy causing difficulties with breathing and causing hypoxia
- Associated medical conditions:
  - obesity
  - diabetes mellitus
  - hypertension
  - hypernatraemia
  - hypokalaemia
- Poor wound healing secondary to high levels of circulating corticosteroids

Why are patients with acromegaly high-risk surgical candidates?

- Anaesthetic difficulties due to problems with face-mask ventilation and intubation as a result of enlargement of the tongue, pharyngeal and laryngeal tissues and distorted facial anatomy
- Associated medical conditions:
  - hypertension
  - diabetes mellitus

- impaired left ventricular function
- sleep apnoea

What are the principles of surgery in a patient with phaeochrocytoma?

Phaechrocytomas are catecholamine producing tumours of the nervous system. Clinical symptoms include headache, hypertension, palpitations and tachycardia. They should be surgically excised under alpha adrenoreceptor (phenoxybenzamine) blockade followed by beta blockade (propanolol), which are given pre-operatively. In the perioperative period, invasive monitoring of central venous and arterial pressures is mandatory. Post-operatively, patients should continue to receive invasive monitoring in ICU with particular attention to fluid balance and glycaemic control.

What are the principles of surgery in a patient with carcinoid syndrome?

These are tumours which secrete 5-HT, kinins, kallikreins, prostaglandins, substance P and histamine. Clinical features include sweating, GI symptoms, hyper- or hypo-tension, and bronchospasm. During surgical excision, somatostatin analogues (octreotide), 5-HT antagonists (methysergide) and antihistamines are given preoperatively. In the perioperative period, invasive monitoring of central venous and arterial pressures is mandatory. Post-operatively, patients should continue to receive invasive monitoring in ICU with particular attention to fluid balance.

F

■ Fluid Management

What are the daily fluid and electrolyte maintenance requirements in an adult?

	Per kg body weight (mmol)	Total for 70 kg adult (mmol)
Na^+	1–2	70–140
K^+	1	70
Cl^-	1	70
PO_4	0.2	14
Ca^+	0.1	7
Mg^+	0.1	7
Water	35 ml	2500 ml

What is the normal daily fluid loss?
- Urine: 1500 ml
- Faeces: 100 ml
- Insensible losses: lung 500 ml; skin 500 ml

What is the effect of surgery on fluid and electrolyte homeostasis?
- ADH released which increases water resorption
- Aldosterone secretion which causes Na^+ retention and K^+ excretion
- K^+ tends to rise due to:
  - cellular injury
  - reduced renal clearance (transient renal impairment common in the immediate post-operative period)
  - blood transfusions

F 121

What is the composition of commonly used fluid preparations?

(mmol l^{-1})	Fluid preparation			
	0.9% saline	5% dextrose	Dextrose (4%) saline (0.18%)	Hartmann's solution
Na$^+$	155	0	30	131
K$^+$	0	0	0	5
Ca$^+$	0	0	0	2
Cl$^-$	155	0	30	111
HCO$_3^-$	0	0	0	29
Glucose	0	278	222	0
Distribution in body water	ECF	ECF	$^1/_2$ ECF; $^1/_2$ ICF	ECF

What is the daily composition of gastrointestinal secretions?

(mmol l^{-1})	Gastrointestinal secretion			
	Gastric	Bile	Pancreatic	Small bowel
Na$^+$	30–80	130	130	130
K$^+$	5–20	10	10	10
Cl$^-$	100–150	100	75	90–130
H$^+$ / HCO$_3^-$	40–60 (H$^+$)	30–50 (HCO$_3^-$)	70–100 (HCO$_3^-$)	20–40 (HCO$_3^-$)
Volume (ml)	2500	500	1000	5000

How do you calculate fluid requirements in the post-operative patient?

- Pre-operative fluid deficit: if pre-surgical fluid resuscitation was not adequate +
- Intra-operative loss: (calculated from amount of fluid/blood collected from sucker bottles, weight of gauze swabs, volume of NGT aspirates, intra-operative urine output) +

- Maintenance requirement (urinary and insensible losses) +
- On-going losses (fistula, drain, diarrhoea, NGT, stoma, ileus)

What are the common daily maintenance regimes for a 70 kg adult?

- 1 litre 0.9% N/saline + 20 mmol K^+ over 8 h
  1 litre 5% Dextrose + 20 mmol K^+ over 8 h
  1 litre 5% Dextrose + 20 mmol K^+ over 8 h

This provides: 3 litres of water; 155 mmol Na^+; 60 mmol K^+

- 1 litre Dextrose saline + 20 mmol K^+ over 8 h
  1 litre Dextrose saline + 20 mmol K^+ over 8 h
  1 litre Dextrose saline + 20 mmol K^+ over 8 h

This provides: 3 litres of water; 90 mmol Na^+; 60 mmol K^+
(safer in first 24h post-surgery when there is Na^+ retention)

- 1 litre Hartmann's solution + 20 mmol K^+ over 8 h
  1 litre 5% Dextrose + 20 mmol K^+ over 8 h
  1 litre 5% Dextrose + 20 mmol K^+ over 8 h

This provides: 3 litres of water; 131 mmol Na^+; 65 mmol K^+

■ Fracture Management I: Basic Principles

Define fracture stability
The lack of movement between fracture fragments. It can be absolute (when there is no motion between the fracture fragments under a physiological load) or relative (when there is some motion between the fracture fragments).

What are the basic principles in the management of any closed fracture?
To achieve:
- union
- alignment
- function

How may this be achieved?
- Non-operatively:
  - analgesia
  - bed rest
  - traction
  - slings
  - splints
  - plaster casts
- Operatively:
  - internal fixation
  - external fixation

What are the indications for internal fixation of fractures?
- Absolute:

- adequate reduction can not be achieved by closed methods
- displaced intra-articular fractures
- non-unions
- major avulsion fractures where there has been loss of function of a joint or muscle group
- Relative:
  - delayed unions
  - multiple fractures
  - pathological fractures
  - elderly patients: to allow early mobilisation
  - fractures with associated neurovascular injury

List the types of implants used in internal fixation
- Those that achieve absolute stability:
  - screws
  - plates
- Those that achieve relative stability:
  - Kirschner wires
  - intramedullary nails

What are the indications for external fixation?
- Temporary stabilisation:
  - to achieve haemorrhage control for pelvic fractures
  - of fractures during life-saving surgery
  - of soft tissue injuries
- Definitive management for:
  - some open fractures
  - some rotationally unstable pelvic fractures
  - non-union of fractures
  - limb lengthening surgery
- To supplement internal fixation

What are the complications following a fracture?

Immediate:
- Neurovascular injury
- Local visceral injury
- Compartment syndrome
- Haemorrhage

Early:
- Wound infection
- Fat embolism
- Exacerbation of existing illness
- ARDS

Late:
- Delayed union because of:
  - poor blood supply
  - severe soft tissue damage
  - infection
  - periosteal stripping
  - inadequate splintage: excessive traction or movement at the fracture site will delay ossification in the callus
  - over-rigid fixation
- Non-union
  - hypertrophic: osteogenesis is still active but not capable of bridging the fracture gap; bone ends are enlarged
  - atrophic: osteogenesis has ceased; bone ends are rounded or tapered with no suggestion of new bone formation
- Malunion because the:
  - fracture was never reduced and has united in an unsatisfactory position
  - fracture was reduced but reduction was not held during healing
  - fracture gradually collapsed during healing of communited or osteoporotic bone

- Fibrous union: excessive movement of the bone ends, which unite by fibrous tissue. Differentiation of synovial cells can lead to a psuedoarthrosis
- Avascular necrosis: bone necrosis occurs after injury. Most commonly affected regions are the femoral head (after fracture of femoral neck or hip dislocation); proximal part of the scaphoid (following scaphoid waist fracture); the lunate (following a fracture or dislocation) and the body of the talus (after fracture of its neck)
- Growth disturbance: in children, damage to the physis may lead to abnormal or arrested growth of the bone
- Joint instability: bone loss or malunion close to a joint may lead to instability or recurrent dislocation
- Osteoarthritis: fractures which damage the articular cartilage can give rise to post-traumatic osteoarthritis
- Soft tissue complications:
  - myositis ossificans: seen especially after fractures around the elbow
  - muscle contracture: sites most commonly involved are the forearm, hand, leg and foot
  - tendon rupture, e.g. extensor pollicus longus tendon after distal radius fracture
  - nerve entrapment: common sites are the median nerve after fractures around the wrist and ulnar nerve after post-traumatic valgus deformity of the elbow
- Complex regional pain syndrome: initially pain is accompanied by swelling, erythema, warmth, tenderness and moderate stiffness of nearby joints; later the skin becomes pale, atrophic with severely restricted movements

■ Fracture Management II: Open Fractures

Classify open fractures

The Gustillo and Anderson classification is the most commonly used in clinical practice.

- Grade 1:   <1 cm clean wound, with a simple fracture pattern
- Grade 2:   >1 cm wound and a low energy fracture pattern
- Grade 3:   high energy crush injuries with extensive muscle damage
- Grade 3A: adequate bone coverage by local soft tissues
- Grade 3B: soft tissue loss over the bone with some contamination or periosteal stripping, which requires a local or free tissue transfer
- Grade 3C: arterial injury requiring repair associated with any fracture pattern

---

Describe the initial management of open fractures in the casualty department

- Deal with primary survey according to ATLS® guidelines
- Control external haemorrhage with direct pressure over the wound
- Opioid analgesia
- Oxygenation and intravenous fluids
- Rapid evaluation of wound
  - remove gross contaminants
  - swab the wound
  - photograph the wound

- cover with moist (betadine or saline) sterile dressing
- Evaluate and record neurovascular status of limb
- Reduce and splint the fracture: re-evaluate and record neurovascular status of limb
- Obtain at least two radiographs of the fracture (which must include the joints above and below the fracture)
- Tetanus toxoid if indicated
- Intravenous antibiotics (usually cephalosporin $\pm$ metronidazole)
- Consult plastic surgical team (should be done before any operative intervention)
- Make arrangements for patient to be taken to operating theatre as soon as possible

Describe the subsequent management of open fractures

Surgical management should commence within 6 hours of injury. It should be managed by a senior orthopaedic surgeon. Surgery should be performed under general anaesthesia and should include:
- Cleaning of the wound:
  - removal of all obvious contaminants
  - skin scrubbed with a brush
  - wound irrigation with at least 9 litres of warm isotonic solution using pulse lavage
- Debridement of:
  - skin edges
  - all tissues of doubtful viability
  - bone which has no soft tissue attachment
- Fracture stabilisation
  - temporary
  - permanent

Should open wounds be left open or closed?

They must be left open and packed with moist dressings. The wound should be re-assessed, in the operating room at 24–48 hours. Ideally, primary closure should be achieved within 5 days of injury.

■ Fracture Healing

Describe the normal phases of fracture healing

Inflammatory phase (time of injury to 24–72 h)

- Haematoma formation: bleeding occurs from vessels within bone, periosteum and adjacent soft tissue. A haematoma and fibrin clot forms, which is a source of haemopoietic cells which secrete growth factors which in turn recruit fibroblasts, mesenchymal cells and osteoprogenitor cells to the fracture site
- Demolition phase: a local inflammatory response ensues with neutrophils, macrophages and mast cells appearing to phagocytose blood clot and tissue debris. Osteoclasts remove dead bone fragments
- Granulation tissue formation: as fibroblasts proliferate, granulation tissue begins to form between the bone ends by ingrowth of capillary loops from below the periosteum and from the fractured bone ends

Reparative phase (48 h to 2 weeks):

- Neovascularisation and local vasodilatation: mediated by vocative substances, e.g. nitric oxide
- Organisation: fracture haematoma is organised; fibroblasts and chondroblasts appear between the bone ends and cartilage is formed (Type II collagen)
- Callus formation: rapid proliferation of osteoprogenitor cells from the inner layer of the cut periosteum and endosteum occurs within 24 h. These cells differentiate into osteoblasts, which form osteoid and chondrocytes, which produce cartilage. Osteoid is mineralised to form woven bone. Callus formed at each side of the fracture then advances towards each other to bridge the fracture site. This is known as the

provisional callus and provides a splint-like supportive function 5–15 days after the injury. The amount of callus formed depends on the anatomical site, the degree of immobilisation and on blood supply. The amount of cartilage formed in the provisional callus varies but is promoted by poor blood supply and by shearing stresses. Within 14–21 days, phagocytic osteoclasts start to remove the woven bone accompanied by orderly lamellar bone synthesis by osteoblasts

Remodelling phase (middle of repair phase up to 5 years):

- The subperiosteal and medullary callus is reconstructed with lamellar bone along lines of mechanical stress to restore full strength and allows bone to assume its normal configuration and shape based on the stresses it is exposed to. Fracture healing is complete when there is repopulation of the medullary canal
- In cortical bone, remodelling occurs by invasion of an osteoclast 'cutting cone', which is then followed by osteoblasts which lay down new lamellar bone (osteon)
- In cancellous bone, remodelling occurs on the surface of the trabeculae, which causes the trabeculae to become thicker

What factors influence fracture healing?

Local factors:

- Degree of local trauma/soft tissue/bone loss
- Infection
- Soft tissue interposition
- Degree of immobilisation/stability
- Local pathological condition
- Vascular supply
- Anatomic location and type of bone fractured
- Degree of immobilisation/stability

Systemic factors:
- Age
- Co-morbidity
- Hormones
  - cortisone decreases callus volume
  - growth hormone and androgens increase callus volume
- Drugs (NSAIDs, corticosteroids)
- Nutrition
  - vitamin C deficiency: depression of collagen biosynthesis
  - vitamin D deficiency: abundant callus formation but fails to calcify
- Cigarette smoke

■ General Anaesthetics

What are the basic principles of achieving general anaesthesia?

- Induction of anaesthesia: usually with intravenous agents, e.g. thiopentone, propofol or etomidate. These agents are highly lipid soluble and rapidly cross the blood brain barrier and hence have a rapid onset of action. They are rapidly redistributed from the brain and thus work for only a short duration
- Maintenance of anaesthesia: usually with inhalational agents, e.g. halothane, isoflurane or enflurane. These are lipid soluble hydrocarbons which have a longer duration of action
- Muscle relaxation: important in many surgical procedures and is achieved with:
  - depolarising agents
  - non-depolarising agents
- Analgesia

List the adverse effects of general anaesthetic agents

- Respiratory
  - airway obstruction
  - ventilatory depression
  - bronchodilatation
- Cardiovascular
  - reduced myocardial contractility
  - decreased cardiac output
  - hypotension
  - arrhythmias
- Central nervous system

- increased intracranial pressure
- increased cerebral blood flow

What is rapid sequence induction?

It is a method of achieving rapid induction of anaesthesia (using thiopentone and suxamethonium) in emergency situations especially when the patient is not fasted and surgery cannot be delayed. Digital cricoid pressure is used to prevent aspiration until tracheal intubation has been accomplished.

What parameters must be monitored in all anaesthetised patients?

- Respiratory:
  - inspired O_2 (Fi O_2)
  - pulse oximetry
  - end- tidal CO_2
- Cardiovascular:
  - heart rate
  - blood pressure
  - ECG
  - invasive blood pressure monitoring (usually only in major surgery)
  - central venous pressure (usually only in major surgery)
- Temperature

What effects do general anaesthetics have on the core body temperature?

They cause hypothermia due to their vasodilatory effects. Radiation of body heat and evaporation from open body cavities along with administration of cold intravenous fluids reduce the temperature further. Heat loss can be minimised by using warming blankets (bear huggers), infusing warm fluids and using warm fluids to irrigate body cavities.

List the possible causes of failure to spontaneously breathe after general anaesthesia

- Airway difficulties due to:
  - obstruction
- Breathing difficulties due to:
  - central depression as a result of residual anaesthetic agents or opiates
  - hypoxia
  - hypercarbia
  - pneumothorax
- Circulatory failure

■ Genes

What are genes?

Genes are units of heredity and represent segments of DNA. All proteins are encoded in DNA and, by definition, the unit of DNA which codes for a protein is a gene. They are transmitted to offspring in gametes, usually as part of a chromosome. The vast majority of genes consist of alternating protein coding segments (exons) and non-protein coding segments (introns) whose function is unknown. Each gene is characterised by a start and termination codon. Activation of genes is subject to a promoter upstream of the gene, which in turn is modulated by an enhancer sequence. The promoter is involved in the attachment of RNA polymerase to the DNA sense strand resulting in transcription of messenger RNA. Translation of the mRNA subsequently occurs on ribosomes found in the cytoplasm. Each codon on the mRNA is recognised by a matching transfer RNA, which contributes its amino acid to the end of the growing protein chain. Most proteins subsequently undergo post-translational processing before becoming biologically active.

Which types of genes are associated with cancers?

Two types of genes show distinctive and apparent causal changes in cancer:

- Proto-oncogenes: these are a group of entirely normal cellular genes concerned with the regulation of normal cellular growth. Proto-oncogenes can be activated to become abnormal modulators of cell proliferation, i.e. oncogenes by:

- point mutation or transactivation of adjacent DNA caused by chemical carcinogens or ionising radiation
- amplification as a result of chromosomal translocation placing the proto-oncogene under the influence of a transcriptional enhancer
- viral integration resulting in insertion of strong viral transcriptional enhancers next to a proto-oncogene
- Oncosuppressor genes: these are genes whose expression appears to prevent neoplasia. Affected individuals inherit one defective copy of the gene. Malignant tumours develop from cells, which lose the residual normal copy by virtue of a second genetic event, the result of spontaneous mutation or exposure to a carcinogen. Examples include:
  - familial retinoblastoma; tumour susceptibility has been traced to the RB-1 gene which lies within chromosome band 13q14
  - familial adenomatous polyposis; APC gene lies within chromosome 5q21

A locus frequently lost in a wide variety of tumours is on the short arm of chromosome 17 (17p13). The oncosuppressor at this site codes for a protein called p53, which is responsible for apoptosis.

■ Grafts and Flaps

What is a reconstructive ladder?

It is a systemic approach to the reconstruction of tissues in order to restore normal structure and function. It involves starting with the simplest solution first and, if this is not plausible, then moving on to the next more complex solution. Starting with the simplest solution the ladder comprises:

- wound dressing
- direct closure
- skin graft
- local flap
- free flap

List the advantages and disadvantages of split-thickness skin grafts

Advantages:

- large wound defects can be covered
- can take on wounds that are contaminated or have a poor blood supply
- conform to irregular contours

Disadvantages:

- less durable and provide less support than full-thickness grafts
- contract in the long-term resulting in poor functional and cosmetic outcome
- can have a different texture and colour compared with the surrounding skin
- donor site morbidity

List the advantages and disadvantages of full-thickness skin grafts

Advantages:

- have the same texture and colour compared with the surrounding skin
- do not contract in the long term
- less donor site morbidity compared with split-thickness grafts
- in children, the graft will grow with the child

Disadvantages:

- not suitable for large wound defects
- donor site often requires a split-thickness graft for closure

What are the common donor sites for split and full thickness skin grafts?

Split thickness grafts can be obtained from almost anywhere in the body but the most commonly used sites are the thighs, proximal arm and volar aspect of the forearm.

Full thickness grafts are obtained depending on the area to be grafted, e.g.

- the upper eyelids for lower eyelid defects
- behind the ear or the neck for defects on the face

Describe the different ways in which a local flap can be performed

- Advancement flap: a flap is formed and stretched forwards to fill the defect
- Rotation flap: a flap is moved sideways into a triangular defect (defect can be made triangular if necessary) leaving no secondary defect
- Transposition flap: similar to a rotation flap but a secondary defect is formed which may require a split-thickness skin graft to repair

What is a free flap?

It is a graft that is transferred to another part of the body along with its artery and vein which are anastomosed to the recipient site. The flap can comprise a single type of tissue or a combination of tissues including skin, fat, deep fascia, muscle and bone.

Give some examples of free flaps

- Skin and facia from the dorsal aspect of the forearm (based on radial artery and accompanying veins)
- Latissimus dorsi muscle flap (based on thoracodorsal vessels) for major limb defects or breast reconstruction
- Transverse rectus abdominis musculo-cutaneous (TRAM) flap (based on inferior epigastric vessels) for breast reconstruction after mastectomy
- Fibula as a vascularised bone graft for jaw reconstructions

What are the reasons for graft failure?

- Infection or contamination (split thickness grafts can withstand minimal contamination)
- Haematoma between graft and wound
- Seroma between graft and wound
- Movement between graft and wound (can be prevented by fixing the graft with sutures or staples)

■ Gunshot and Blast Wounds

Should ballistic wounds be classified according to missile velocity?

No. Velocity is not important as the amount of kinetic energy transferred to tissues and therefore ballistic wounds should be classified according to the energy transferred to the tissues, i.e. low-energy or high-energy. Kinetic energy transfer is dependent on missile velocity, presenting area of fragment and mechanical properties of tissue.

How do fragment injuries differ from those caused by bullets?

Fragments injuries are typically small, numerous with a low velocity and low energy transfer. Poor tissue penetration means that the injury is most frequently limited to the path of the missile.

Damage caused by bullet injuries is dependent on the type of firearm used:

- Airguns fire a small, blunt pellet which poorly infiltrates tissue but can cause eyeball injuries or pneumothorax
- Shotguns propel a large number of lead pellets and the depth of tissue penetration is dependent upon the distance from the gun. At close range, widespread tissue damage and skin burns occur. The entry wound appears as a single small hole and an exit wound is rare. At longer distances, the pellets are scattered over a larger area
- Handguns usually fire a large bullet at a relatively low velocity with a low energy transfer and so result in localised damage to the structures directly in the path of the missile

- Rifle bullets are of high velocity with a high energy transfer and so cause extensive damage. The high-energy transfer from the bullet to the surrounding tissues causes a large cavity to be formed along the track which finishes in a large exit wound

How do bullets cause tissue damage?
- Directly: in low energy transfer wounds damage is caused from direct effects along the path of the bullet
- Indirectly: in high energy transfer wounds indirect effects are responsible for the damage caused
- By yaw: rifle bullets tumble (yaw) within the wound, increasing the wound track and maximising tissue damage and increasing the surface area that the bullet presents to the tissues
- By cavitation: as a bullet infiltrates a wound a temporary cavity is created which in turn produces a vacuum and sucks in debris and other contaminants. In high-energy wounds, tissue damage including bone fractures can occur far away from the wound pathway as a result of cavitation

How do blast injuries differ from those caused by missiles?
- Bullet injuries tend to damage fluid-filled organs (liver, kidney, spleen, brain and bone) rather than air-filled organs (lung, bowel). In blast injuries, compressive forces cause damage to air-filled structures rather than fluid filled organs
- In blast injuries, the blast wave can be trapped within a confined compartment, so the extent of injury may be magnified greatly
- Blast waves can compress victims resulting in significant tissue damage, visceral rupture, haemorrhage and increased compartment pressures

- Blast injuries produce secondary damage from fragments produced from surrounding structures or fires
- Blast winds can displace victims, throwing the body or causing structures to collapse onto them
- Blast injuries are associated with specific injuries, e.g. tympanic membrane rupture, lung injuries (blast lung), air embolism and crush injuries

■ Head Injury

What do you understand by the terms primary and secondary head injuries?

Primary injury: insult caused to the brain at the time of impact. It is caused by shearing forces, which tear axonal tracts. The damage caused can be diffuse or focal. There is no treatment and the focus of intervention is to prevent secondary complications.

Secondary injury: occurs due to hypoxia (from obstructed airway or impaired respiratory drive), hypotension (from associated injuries) and raised intracranial pressure (due to haematoma, oedema, infection or abscess).

What is the initial management of the patient with a head injury?

Patients should be managed according to ATLS® principles:
- Airway protection with C-spine immobilisation
- Ensure adequacy of breathing
- Maintain circulation and control haemorrhage
- Assessment of the severity of head injury using the Glasgow Coma Score (GCS)

What are the indications for a CT scan?
- GCS < 13 at any stage since injury or 2 h post-injury
- Focal neurological deficit
- Persistent confusion
- Any skull fracture
- Seizures following injury
- Amnesia

- Difficulty in assessing patient, e.g. due to alcohol
- Penetrating skull injury

What are the indications for a skull radiograph?
Same indications as for a CT, if scanning facilities are not available.

What are the criteria for admission following a head injury?
- Abnormality detected on CT scan
- Fluctuating GCS despite absence of abnormalities on a CT scan
- Patients on anticoagulant therapy

What are the indications for referral to a neurosurgeon?
- Presence of any intracranial bleeding
- GCS < 8 despite adequate resuscitation
- Confusion > 8 h post-injury
- Progressive neurological deficit
- Compound skull fractures
- A child with a tense fontanelle

What are the indications for intubation?
- GCS $\leq$ 8
- GCS 9–12 and patient is being transferred to another centre
- Uncontrolled seizures
- Loss of cough or gag reflex
- Respiratory compromise

What are the criteria for intracranial pressure monitoring?
- Head injury induced coma
- Patients with severe head injuries who require surgery for associated injuries

- Patients who require prolonged ventilation for pulmonary injuries

What are the risks of an intracranial haematoma in patients with head injuries?
- No skull fracture
  - patient orientated   1 : 6000
  - patient not orientated   1 : 120
- Skull fracture
  - patient orientated   1 : 32
  - patient not orientated   1 : 4

What are the possible complications following a head injury?
- Epilepsy
- Meningitis and cerebral abscesses
- Amnesia
- Post-concussional syndrome (headache, dizziness, poor concentration, memory impairment, behavioural changes)
- Chronic subdural haematoma
- Hydrocephalus
- Peptic ulceration
- Diabetes incipidus/SIADH
- Disseminated intravascular coagulation
- Encephalopathy (mainly in repeated head injuries, e.g. in boxers)

■ HIV/Hepatitis and Surgery

What precautions should be taken when operating on patients with hepatitis and HIV?

- Minimise the number of theatre staff
- All skin breaks on the surgeon should be dressed with waterproof dressing
- Only vital equipment to be left in theatre
- Use tourniquets when possible to minimise bleeding
- Use disposable equipment whenever possible
- Double gloving
- Disposable impervious gowns and drapes
- Face visors
- Close supervision of inexperienced staff
- Minimise use of sharp instruments whenever possible
- No hand-to-hand passing of instruments
- Only a single operator's hands within a wound, where possible
- Theatre to be thoroughly cleaned following the procedure

What is the management of occupational exposure to these viruses?

- Hepatitis B:
  - unvaccinated personnel should receive HBV hyperimmune globulin within 24 h of exposure and recombinant HBV vaccine within the next 7 days
  - test antibody levels at 4–6 months after administration of immune globulin and vaccination
  - personnel should be advised on ways to prevent transmission to their patients, household contacts and sexual partners

- referral to specialist medical care for those found to have seroconverted
- Hepatitis C:
  - post-exposure prophylaxis with immune globulin no longer recommended
  - test immediately after exposure (serum saved) and 6–9 months later to detect antibodies and to look for evidence of hepatitis
  - personnel should be advised on ways to prevent transmission to their patients, household contacts and sexual partners
  - regular testing of the employee for hepatitis
  - referral to specialist medical care
  - antiviral therapy maybe offered for chronic HCV infection
- HIV:
  - If chemoprophylaxis to be given, it should be initiated within 1 h of exposure
  - 24 h access to advice on prophylaxis and support for stress associated with the situation
  - regular testing of the employee for HIV
  - personnel should be advised on ways to prevent transmission to their patients, household contacts and sexual partners

■ Immune System

How can the immune system be classified?

- Non-specific defences:
  - mechanical: e.g. skin, epithelium
  - humoral fluids: secreted by most body tissues, e.g. gastric acid, pancreatic enzymes, sebum
  - cellular: neutrophils, eosinophils, macrophages, mast cells, complement system
- Specific immunity: dependent on lymphocytes. Antibodies are produced by B-lymphocytes whilst the cellular immune responses are initiated by T-lymphocytes. B-lymphocytes undergo maturation in bone marrow whereas T-lymphocytes do so in the thymus. In response to a specific stimulus a clone of activated lymphocytes are produced. In the case of B-lymphocytes, the effector cells are antibody-producing plasma cells. In the T-cell system, a variety of effector cells including cytotoxic, helper and suppressor T-cells are produced. In addition, clonal proliferation of B- and T-cells results in populations of antigen specific memory cells

Briefly describe the structure of immunoglobulins

All immunoglobulins are composed of two heavy chains and two light chains; the heavy chains arranged in parallel centrally with a shorter light chain on either side. Heavy chains differ structurally for each class of immunoglobulin with the letters gamma, mu, alpha, delta and epsilon used to indicate the heavy chains of IgG, IgM, IgA, IgD and IgE, respectively. The C-terminal end of the heavy chains is constant (known as the Fc piece). This part of the molecule is bound by disulphide bonds which can be cleaved by papain or pepsin at specific sites. There are only two types of light chain (kappa and lambda) in all classes and each molecule will have one or the other. The N-terminal ends of the heavy and light chains are highly variable and constitute the specific antigen binding site (Fab).

What is the structure and function of the different immunoglobulins?

- IgG: monomer; binds to macrophages and neutrophils; involved in complement activation and secondary response; undergoes placental transfer; most abundant immunoglobulin in plasma and extravascular space
- IgM: pentamer; involved in primary response and complement activation; B-cell antigen receptor
- IgA: monomer and dimeric; principal immunoglobulin produced at mucosal surfaces
- IgE: monomer; bound to mast cells by its Fc fragment; involved in Type 1 immediate hypersensitivity reactions
- IgD: monomer; has a B-cell antigen receptor

Immune Deficiency and Surgery

Classify the causes of immune deficiency

Primary: rare and manifest in childhood; they can be due to:

- complement deficiencies
- phagocytosis deficiencies
- T-cell defects, e.g. DiGeorge's syndrome: selective T-cell deficiency resulting in failure of the third and fourth branchial arches to develop. The thymus, parathyroids, some parafollicular cells in the thyroid and the ultimobranchial body fails to develop. Affected infants have total absence of cell-mediated immune responses; they can deal with pyogenic bacteria infections but not with opportunistic infections such as *Pneumocystis carinii*, fungal or viral infections. Live vaccine inoculation may be fatal
- B-cell defects, e.g. Bruton-type α, α-globulinaemia; due to failure in maturation of B-cells within the bone marrow resulting in virtual absence of serum immunoglobulins. Recurrent pyogenic infections occur in infancy once maternal IgG has been catabolised
- combined immunodeficiency syndromes: heterogeneous group of disorders such as 'Swiss Type' and ataxic telangiectasia. There is gross functional impairment of T- and B-cell-mediated immune function; patients usually die within 2 years from overwhelming recurrent sepsis

Secondary (acquired): these are conditions in which the immune system develops and functions normally but becomes defective as a result of:

- immunosuppressive therapy
- chemotherapy
- radiotherapy
- malignancy
- splenectomy
- HIV/AIDS
- diabetes mellitus
- major surgery
- trauma
- infection
- malnutrition

Why should surgeons know something about immunodeficiency disorders?

- Common surgical conditions occur in immunocompromised patients
- Signs of surgical disease (e.g. peritonitis) may be masked in immunocompromised patients
- Some surgical conditions are more common in patients taking immunosuppressive therapy:
  - peptic ulceration, pancreatitis and diverticular disease in patients taking corticosteroids
  - pseudomembranous colitis in patients receiving frequent courses of antibiotics
- Immunodeficient patients are at greater risk of developing certain surgical conditions:
  - small bowel lymphoma
  - intra-abdominal abscesses
  - neutropenic colitis
  - CMV enterocolitis
- Morbidity and mortality rates are higher following surgery in immunocompromised patients

What are the principles of surgery in immunocompromised patients?

- Pre-operative:
  - fluid resuscitation with correction of any electrolyte disturbances
  - correction of any nutritional deficiencies
  - optimisation of underlying disease
  - antibiotic prophylaxis
  - doses of immunosuppressive therapy may need to be changed and/or administered intravenously
  - in renal transplant patients, avoid blood pressure cuffs being applied to an arm in which an AV fistula is sited
- Operative:
  - meticulous surgical technique and haemostasis as these patients have a low immunological capacity to cope with infected haematomas
  - avoid use of drains, wherever possible
  - stomas should be considered rather than anastomosis as leaks are poorly tolerated
- Post-operative:
  - antibiotic prophylaxis to avoid wound infections
  - minimal handling of wounds
  - early removal of drains, urinary catheters and central venous catheters
  - sutures and ligatures should be retained for longer than normal
  - regular examination of patients to identify possible infective complications
  - regular microbiological observation with swabs taken from wounds and drain sites; blood, urine and sputum should be sent for culture analysis if infection suspected

■ Jaundice

How is jaundice classified?

Into pre-hepatic, hepatic and post-hepatic (obstructive)
causes

	Pre-hepatic	Hepatic	Post-hepatic
Causes	Haemolysis Spherocytosis Gilbert disease Crigler–Najar syndrome	Hepatitis Cirrhosis: alcoholic, primary, biliary Drugs Liver tumours: primary, secondary	Gallstones Atresia Stricture Pancreatitis Pancreatic tumours Cholangiocarcinoma Cysts Parasitic infection
Bilirubin	Unconjugated	Conjugated or unconjugated	Conjugated
Urine colour	Normal	Dark	Dark
Stool colour	Normal	Normal	Pale
Serum ALP	Normal	Mildly raised (high in PBC)	Very high
Serum amino-transferase	Normal	Very high	Normal/slightly raised
Prothrombin time	Normal	Prolonged: not correctable with vitamin K	Prolonged: correctable with vitamin K

How should a jaundiced patient be assessed?

- Clinical history:
  - hepatitis: recent travel, recreational drug use, joint pains
  - gallstones: fat intolerance, recurrent RUQ pain

- haemolytic disorders: tendency to bruising, family history of bleeding disorders
- obstructive jaundice: pale stool, dark urine
- cirrhosis: alcohol abuse
- malignancy: anorexia, weight loss
- hepatocellular damage: drug history (phenothiazines, methyltestosterone)
- Physical examination:
  - jaundice
  - chronic liver disease: spider naevi, ascites, palmar erythema, finger clubbing, painful hepatomegaly
  - malignancy: painless hepatomegaly, palpable gall bladder (*Courvoisier's law*)
- Laboratory studies:
  - FBC: anaemia, increased reticulocyte count (haemolysis), raised WCC (cholangitis)
  - blood film: (sickle cells, spherocytes)
  - clotting: increased prothrombin time
  - liver studies: bilirubinuria, raised serum bilirubin, raised ALP (obstructive causes), increased AST/ALT (hepatitis), raised gamma GT (alcohol), low albumin
- Urine/stool analysis:
  - bilirubin in urine (obstructive causes)
  - excess urobilinogen in urine (pre-hepatic or hepatic causes)
  - absence of urobilinogen in urine (obstructive causes)
  - raised faecal urobilinogen (pre-hepatic causes)
  - absence of bile pigments in stools (hepatic or obstructive causes)
- Radiology:
  - AXR: 10% of gallstones are radio-opaque; calcification in chronic pancreatitis; air cholangiogram; enlarged gallbladder (soft tissue mass in RUQ)

- Ultrasound: allows assessment of liver texture, gall bladder for stones and CBD diameter (normal CBD diameter <6 mm unless previous ERCP, cholecystectomy or age >65 years). Not reliable for stones within the CBD as often obscured by gas in the duodenum. Ultrasound also allows confirmation of the presence of ascites
  - CT: useful if USS findings equivocal or for staging of tumours
  - MRCP: non-invasive and safer than ERCP
- Radionuclide scanning: allows imaging of the biliary tree
- ERCP: allows biopsy or brush cytology, stone extraction or stenting
- Histology: liver biopsy but check clotting times first

Describe the peri-operative management of obstructive jaundice?

- Pre-operative biliary decompression: improves post-operative outcome
- Broad spectrum antibiotic prophylaxis
- Parenteral vitamin K +/− fresh frozen plasma
- Pre-operative iv fluid administration with careful monitoring of fluid balance (urinary catheter ± CVP monitoring)

What are the risks of surgery in the jaundiced patient?

- Bleeding: the liver is responsible for manufacture of clotting factors in the intrinsic and extrinsic clotting pathways. Vitamin K-dependent factors (II, VII, IX and X) are not manufactured in obstructive jaundice as Vitamin K is a lipid and dependent on normal bile excretion.
  Additionally, the presence of portal hypertension may result in significant haemorrhage
- Cholangitis: develops in the presence of bile duct obstruction and infection. Gram-negative organisms, e.g.

Klebsiella and *E. coli* are the commonest organisms found. Charcot's triad (fever, jaundice and RUQ pain) characterises cholangitis. Jaundice in the absence of cholangitis generally results in poor leukocyte function impairing the body's immune response

- Hepatorenal failure: aetiology not known but possible causes include the combination of relative ischaemia combined with direct toxicity of hyperbilirubinaemia to the nephron or secondary to bacterial toxins
- Wound infection
- Impaired drug metabolism

■ Joint Replacement

What is the aim of any joint replacement?
It is to provide the patient with a pain-free, stable joint that is capable of bearing the loads required whilst allowing an adequate range of movement.

What are the main indications for joint arthroplasty?
- Arthropathies:
  - osteoarthritis
  - rheumatoid arthritis
  - traumatic arthritis
  - juvenile rheumatoid arthritis
- Avascular necrosis
- Fractures
- Tumours
- Metabolic bone disorders

What are the contra-indications to joint replacements?
- Absolute:
  - active infection
- Relative:
  - skeletal immaturity
  - non-ambulators
  - neuropathic joints (Charcot joint)
  - progressive neurological disease
  - muscle weakness around the joint

What are its complications?
- Local risks:
  - limb length inequality

- dislocation
- infection
- nerve injuries
- periprosthetic fracture
- loosening
- Systemic risks:
  - chest infection
  - urinary tract infection
  - deep venous thrombosis
  - pulmonary embolism
  - mortality

What materials are joint replacement implants made of?
- Ultra-high molecular weight polyethylene (UHMWPE)
- Titanium
- Oxynium
- Cobalt-chrome
- Silicone (used as a spacer)

What guidelines should be followed when performing hip and knee arthroplasty?
National Institute of Clinical Excellence (NICE) guidelines, which state that the:
- prosthesis used should have a 10 yr follow-up published in peer-reviewed journals with life table, survivorship curve and with at least 90% 10 yr survival
- hospitals in which the surgery is conducted must have a high dependency and intensive treatment unit (HDU/ITU), dedicated orthopaedic wards with appropriately trained staff and ultra-clean air-dedicated orthopaedic theatres
- prophylactic antibiotics should be given for the first 36 hr in hip replacements and at least at induction for knee replacements

- all patients should have good quality AP and lateral (and 25 degree skyline view for knee replacements) radiographs prior to discharge from hospital
- patients should be followed up with radiographs annually for the first 5 years and every 5 years thereafter

What should preoperative assessment consist of?
- Detailed history to ensure that pain is from the joint and not referred pain
- Systemic examination including examination of the affected joint
- Dental evaluation
- Routine blood tests (including group and save)
- Mid stream urine sample
- Swabs taken to rule out MRSA colonisation
- Recent X-rays of the affected joint in two planes
- Planning of surgical approach and templating

Which factors influence the long-term survival of prosthetic implants?
- Patient factors:
  - underlying diagnosis
  - gender
- Implant factors:
  - type of implant used
  - type of cement used
- Surgical factors:
  - cementing technique
  - surgical approach

■ Laparoscopy

Briefly describe how laparoscopy is performed?

Patient is placed in the Trendeleburgh position. A Veress needle is passed sub-umbilically and pneumoperitoneum created using an insufflator set to deliver 1l of CO_2/min initially, then at 5 l/min until a pressure of 10–12 mmHg is maintained. The Veress needle is removed and a 10 mm trocar with a cannula inserted through the same incision. A 10 mm $0°$ diagnostic laparoscope attached to a video camera is then passed through the cannula. Two 5 mm ports are introduced in the right quadrant, one in the mid-clavicular line and the other in the anterior axillary line. In the open technique, a Hasson cannula is used.

How do you know that the needle is in the peritoneal cavity?

- Passage of fluid without resistance
- Fluid can be aspirated back easily
- Absence of air (presence of air could mean needle is in the bowel!)

What are the potential risks of excessive insufflation?

- Pneumothorax
- DVT (increased intra-thoracic pressure ($\Rightarrow$ reduced venous return from lower limbs))

What are the contraindications to laparoscopic surgery?

- Bleeding diathesis
- Severe adhesions
- Peritonitis

- Pregnancy
- Severe COPD

What are the complications of laparoscopic surgery?
- Perforation of abdominal viscus
- Haemorrhage
- Pneumomediastinum
- Pneumothorax
- Port site hernia
- Sepsis

Large Bowel Obstruction

What are the causes of large bowel obstruction?
- Colorectal carcinoma
- Diverticular disease
- Intussusception
- Volvulus
  - sigmoid: predisposing factors include a high fibre diet, a long mobile sigmoid colon, chronic constipation, elderly patients
  - caecal: usually associated with a congenital malrotation
- Crohn's disease
- Strictures: inflammatory, ischaemic or anastomotic

Why is the ileo-caecal valve of importance in large bowel obstruction?
If the ileo-caecal valve is open, the contents of the large bowel will pass in to the small intestine thus decompressing the large bowel and reducing the risk of perforation. However, if the ileo-caecal valve remains closed, the intraluminal pressure within the caecum will rise rapidly and perforation with faecal peritonitis will occur if the obstruction remains untreated.

What are the clinical features of large bowel obstruction?
- Caecal tumours present with small bowel obstruction: colicky central abdominal pain, abdominal distention, early vomiting and late absolute constipation
- Left-sided tumours present with: change in bowel habit, lower abdominal pain, marked abdominal distention, late vomiting and early absolute constipation

What is the management of large bowel obstruction?

- Patients should be kept nil by mouth with administration of intravenous analgesia and fluids
- Placement of a naso-gastric tube
- Antibiotics to cover gram-negative and anaerobic organisms
- Appropriate investigations:
  - bloods: WCC, U and Es
  - abdominal X-ray: dilated large bowel; dilated small bowel depending on competence of ileo-caecal valve; 'bent inner-tube' sign classical of sigmoid volvulus; grossly dilated caecum often located in the left upper quadrant in caecal volvulus
  - enema with water-soluble contrast (e.g. Gastrograffin)
  - CT with intravenous and rectal contrast

What are the principles of surgery in a patient with large bowel obstruction?

- Relieve the obstruction:
  - using a stent
  - using needle decompression
  - milking intestinal contents back up the NG tube; this procedure should commence from the level of the obstruction or the ileo-caecal junction
  - by milking the bowel contents through the proximal resection margin
  - with on-table lavage
  - with a defunctioning colostomy
- Correct the cause: this may not always be possible at initial surgery; colonoscopic decompression and insertion of a flatus tube should be initially attempted in cases of sigmoid volvulus
- Maintain intestinal continuity: resect non-viable bowel and consider a primary anastomosis

What are the surgical options in the management of acute large bowel obstruction?

- One-stage procedure: intra-operative colonic irrigation, resection of non-viable bowel and primary anastomosis. It avoids a stoma and is useful in elderly patients where a staged procedure is best avoided. Patients will have diarrhoea for 3–4 months post-operatively, after which bowel actions settle down
- Two-stage procedure:
  - bowel resected; proximal end brought out as terminal colostomy and distal end as a mucus fistula or closed as a Hartmann's procedure; 2–3 months post-surgery, end-to-end anastomosis is performed
  - bowel resected and end-to-end anastomosis is performed; defunctioning transverse colostomy or a loop ileostomy is fashioned to protect the anastomosis which is closed 3–4 weeks later
  - colonic stent is inserted to relieve the obstruction and a one-stage resection is performed a few days later
- Three stage procedure: initially a transverse colostomy is performed; 2–3 weeks later, bowel is resected with end to end anastomosis; 4–6 weeks later, the colostomy is closed

What do you understand by the term pseudo-obstruction?

This is a functional obstruction of the large bowel. Aetiology includes post-surgery, trauma, idiopathic, metabolic/electrolyte disturbances, drugs, neuropathies and myopathies. The patients are usually elderly and institutionalised. Clinical features which distinguish it from mechanical obstruction are a gradual onset of abdominal distention with minimal pain, and on examination the abdomen is non-tender, and tympanic with quiet bowel sounds. If diagnosis remains uncertain, an instant gastrograffin enema will confirm the free passage of contrast all the way round to the caecum (in mechanical obstruction, contrast does not flow past the obstructing lesion). Management is usually conservative and includes correction of any electrolyte disturbances; administration of iv fluids with placement of a naso-gastric tube; early decompression with a sigmoidoscope and flatus tube. Neostigmine has been shown to be of some benefit. The condition usually resolves spontaneously within a few days. If conservative treatment fails, consider surgery; options include: caecostomy and resection with end ileostomy with a mucus fistula.

■ Lasers

What is Laser?
Light Amplification by Stimulated Emission of Radiation

How are lasers classified?
According to the amount of damage they can cause:
- Class 1: safe even after unlimited exposure
- Class 2: safe within the time of the blink reflex, e.g. 70 ms
- Class 3: cause blindness after short exposure from mirrored surfaces but not rough surfaces
- Class 4: unsafe even with reflection from non-specular surfaces (all medical lasers belong to Class 4)

What are the characteristics of laser light?
- Collimated: output beam is parallel resulting in minimal energy loss when projected over a long distance
- Coherent: waves are all in phase resulting in minimal energy loss
- Chromacity: all of the same wavelength, i.e. monochromic

Classify lasers
- Solid state: contains crystals which produce light when pumped by flash tubes, e.g. neodymium-YAG
- Liquid state: dye compounds are dissolved in alcohol and can operate at different wavelengths (unlike solid and gas lasers)
- Gas state: depend on electron pumping of mixtures of gases, e.g. argon, CO_2

List some uses of lasers in surgery

• Neodymium-YAG	coagulation of tumours, bleeding ulcers
• Argon	ophthalmology, bleeding ulcers
• CO_2	cutting tissues
• Excimer	photorefractive keratotomy
• Ruby	removal of tattoos

How does laser–tissue interaction occur?

- Photo-chemical: a photosensitive drug which concentrates in rapidly growing cells (e.g. tumours) is given to the patient. Laser is used to target these cells
- Photo-thermal: in diabetic retinopathy, a continuous wave argon laser is used to destroy the peripheral retina. This will reduce the retina's blood supply which in turn will reduce the proliferation of retinal vessels, which would cause blindness
- Photo-mechanical: a pulsed dye laser is used via an optical fibre to break up for example bladder or renal stones
- Photo-ablation: a short pulsed wavelength is used to destroy small areas of tissues, e.g. in photoreactive keratomy

What are the advantages and disadvantages of using laser?

Advantages:
- allows treatment of areas with difficult access
- allows precision cutting of tissues
- minimal damage to adjacent tissues
- cutting can be combined with haemostasis

Disadvantages:
- fire risk if the beam is focused on inflammable objects
- retinal or corneal damage if the beam strikes the eyes
- skin burns to patient or theatre personnel

What precautions should be used when working with lasers?

- They should only be operated by trained personnel
- Use of safety goggles (patient and operator)
- Only necessary theatre staff to remain in the operating room
- Warning sign displayed outside the operating room
- Laser machine should make a warning sound every time it is being fired

■ Latex Allergy

What is latex allergy?
Latex is the milky fluid derived from the lactiferous cells of the rubber tree, *Hevea brasiliens*. Latex allergy is an allergy to the products made from the natural rubber latex.

Describe the pathophysiology of latex allergy
Latex exposure is associated with three clinical syndromes:
- Mechanical disruption of the skin due to rubbing of gloves resulting in irritant dermatitis. This is the most common syndrome, is not immune mediated and does not cause allergic complications
- Delayed type iv hypersensitivity reaction, resulting in contact dermatitis 24–48 h after exposure in a sensitised patient. The dermatitis can predispose patients to further sensitisation or infections
- Type I hypersensitivity reaction whereby following re-exposure to latex in sensitised patients, the antigen binds to IgE antibodies on the surface of basophils and mast cells resulting in the release of inflammatory mediators such as histamine, prostaglandins, kinins, leukotrienes and platelet activating factor. Clinical features can vary from mild (urticaria, rhinitis, hoarseness, abdominal pain, nausea) to life-threatening (bronchospasm, laryngeal oedema, hypotension and cardiovascular collapse) symptoms

Which group of patients are at high risk from latex allergy?
Patients who have:
- a history of atopy

- a history of allergy to balloons, rubber gloves or cross-reactive food products such as bananas, potatoes or tomatoes
- had chronic exposure to latex, e.g. health care professionals, rubber industry workers
- been in contact with latex through repeated urinary catheterisations or multiple surgeries
- spina bifida (incidence up to 40%)

What are the common sources of latex in hospitals?
- Gloves (examination, surgical)
- Monitoring devices (blood pressure cuffs, pulse oximetry, ECG wires)
- Stethoscopes
- Tourniquets
- Catheters
- Intravenous tubing ports
- Syringe plungers
- Electrode pads
- Anaesthetic equipment (oxygen mask, suction catheters, respirators)
- Wound drain and tubes

Which tests are available to diagnose latex allergy?
- Skin prick or patch testing
- Serum testing: radioallergosorbent (RAST), which detects and quantifies IgE antibodies
- Enzyme-linked assay of latex specific IgE (ELISA)

What is the management of the patient with latex allergy undergoing surgery?
- Place latex allergy sign on patient's door and above patient's bed
- Patients should wear a latex allergy bracelet

- Document the allergy on all medical and nursing notes including drug charts
- Use latex-free syringes to prepare medications
- Stockinettes can be used to cover stethoscopes and tubing
- Notify theatres as soon as possible
- Notify the sterile surgical services department so that latex-containing items are not mixed with non-latex items
- Remove all latex-containing items from the operating room and thoroughly clean the theatre the night before surgery
- The patient should be scheduled for the first case of the day
- Change filters in the positive pressure air system
- Intra-operatively avoid the use of latex surgical gloves and latex containing materials coming into contact with the patient
- Inform the recovery room at least 30 min prior to end of surgery to allow them to prepare for the arrival of the patient

■ Limping Child

What is the most common reason for a painful limp in a child?

Trauma, this can range from soft tissue injuries to fractures.

What are the non-traumatic causes of a limp in a child?

These can be summarised according to child's age.

Age 1–5 years:

- transient synovitis of the hip
- septic arthritis of the hip
- Perthe's disease
- late presentation of DDH

Age 5–10 years:

- transient synovitis of the hip
- Perthe's disease
- juvenile chronic arthritis
- septic arthritis of the hip

Age 10–15 years:

- slipped upper femoral epiphysis (SUFE)
- septic arthritis of the hip
- transient synovitis of the hip
- juvenile chronic arthritis

What is transient synovitis?

It is a non-specific transient inflammation of the synovium of the hip joint. It is often caused by a viral infection and the child may give a recent history of upper-respiratory tract, ear or gastro-intestinal infection. An effusion of the hip joint is often present which stretches the capsule and causes pain. The child will prefer to hold the hip flexed, abducted and externally rotated as the tension in the capsule is at its lowest in this position.

Is the child with transient synovitis usually unwell?
No. The child is usually systemically well but may have a flu-like illness.

How may a child with transient synovitis present?
- Pain: may be poorly localised in children
- Limp
- Stiffness
- Reluctance to weight bear
- Reduced range of hip movements on examination

What investigations should be performed before making a diagnosis of transient synovitis?
- Blood tests
  - white cell count (WCC)
  - erythrocyte sedimentation rate (ESR)
  - C-reactive protein (CRP)
  - blood cultures
- Plain X-rays
  - frog-leg lateral is useful for excluding Perthe's disease
- Ultrasound of the hip
  - determines presence of an effusion which can be aspirated if infection is suspected

How can transient synovitis be distinguished from septic arthritis?
From four independent clinical predictors:
- history of fever
- inability to weight bear
- ESR $\geq$ 40 mm/hr
- WCC $>$ 12 000

Number of predictors present	Predicted probability of septic arthritis (%)
0	<0.2
1	3.0
2	40
3	93
4	>99

■ Local Anaesthetics

Classify local anaesthetic agents
- Amides, e.g. lignocaine, bupivicaine, prilocaine or ropivicaine
- Esters, e.g. cocaine

What is their mode of action?
They reversibly block Na^+ channels within nerve cells thereby blocking the transmission of an action potential. Smaller nerve fibres (e.g. unmyelinated C fibres) are more sensitive and increasing doses are required to block fibres transmitting sympathetic pain, temperature, proprioception and motor function. This is known as differential conduction blockade and explains why patients often feel pressure but not pain and hence why a nerve block should be tested prior to surgery.

List their uses
- Nerve blocks
- Field blocks
- Epidural pain relief
- Spinal anaesthesia

List their side effects
- Anaphylaxis
- Cardiovascular:
  - arrhythmias
  - myocardial depression
- Central nervous system:
  - peri-oral tingling
  - anxiety

- light-headedness
- tinnitus
- convulsions
- Respiratory
  - apnoea

List some commonly used local anaesthetics along with their half lives and onset of action

Lignocaine	3 ml/kg	$t_{1/2} = 2$ h	Fast acting
Bupivicaine	3–5 ml/kg	$t_{1/2} = 2$ h	Moderately fast acting
Prilocaine	2 ml/kg	$t_{1/2} = 3$ h	Slow acting

List two drugs that can be used in combination with used local anaesthetics

- Adrenaline: to overcome the vasodilatory effects of local anaesthetics thus prolonging their duration of action and reducing bleeding. Adrenaline should not be used in end arteries
- Opioid analgesics (morphine or fentanyl): to improve the quality of analgesia when given via the spinal or epidural route

How much lignocaine is there in a 1% solution?

10 mg/ml

Why may toxicity develop?

- Drug overdose
- Intravascular injection rather than subcutaneous administration
- Injection into areas with a rich blood supply, e.g. head and neck from where there will be faster absorption into the systemic circulation
- In elderly patients, who have a lower threshold for toxicity

- Patients with liver disease may not be able to metabolise the drug resulting in elevated plasma concentrations

How is toxicity managed?
- Stop drug injection immediately
- Maintain airway: intubation may be required
- Maintain breathing: oxygen ± ventilation
- Maintain circulation: rapid intravenous fluids ± inotropes

■ Minimal Access Surgery

Define minimal access surgery

Minimally Invasive Surgery (MIS) refers to a group of techniques that permit access to the internal organs or joints without the use of a customary large incision.

What are the advantages and disadvantages of minimal access surgery?

Advantages are reduced:

- trauma to tissues
- post-operative pain
- post-operative complications
- recovery time (hence reduced hospital in-stay)
- wound size (with fewer wound complications, less scarring and better cosmesis)

Disadvantages are increased:

- operative time (especially initially as technical skills are learnt)
- cost
- risk of iatrogenic injuries
- difficulty with controlling bleeding
- difficulty with removing bulky organs

List some procedures in which minimal access surgery is well established

- Laparoscopic:
  - cholecystectomy
  - appendicectomy
  - splenectomy
  - fundoplication

- Thoracoscopic:
  - myotomy
  - repair of oesophageal atresia and tracheoesophageal fistula
- Ureteropyeloscopy for treatment of:
  - tumours of the prostate, tumours lining the ureter, small renal tumours
  - ureteral and kidney stones
  - ureteral strictures
- Arthroscopy for:
  - diagnostic purposes
  - therapeutic purposes, e.g. meniscal repairs
  - assisted ACL reconstructions

■ Needles

How are suture needles classified?
- By the type of needle point:
  - blunt point needles (○) have a tapered body with a rounded blunt point to limit splitting of tissues such as the liver or kidney
  - conventional cutting needles (▲) have three cutting edges contained within the first third of the needle shaft with the third edge located on the inside concave curvature of the needle pointing towards the wound. These are general purpose needles designed to pass through dense, irregular and thick tissues
  - reverse-cutting needles (▼) have three cutting edges contained along the whole length of the needle shaft with the third edge located on the outer convex curvature of the needle point. The suture is tied against the hole produced by the needle. These are strong needles which can penetrate tough tissues
  - round-body taper point needles (●) are oval or round in cross-section and pierce rather than cut tissues. The penetrating point is smoothly tapered into the round bodied shaft to produce the smallest possible hole size. They are commonly used in anastomoses
  - taper-cutting needles (▲) have reverse-cutting edge tips, which penetrate tough tissues and a round-body, which prevents cutting into surrounding tissue. They are usually used for tendon repairs
- By their attachment to the suture:
  - swaged needles have the suture attached to the needle base

- eyed needles require the surgeon to thread the suture through the eye of the needle; they are associated with increased tissue trauma
- By shape:
  - straight needles are used for easily accessible tissues
  - curved needles are formed in an arc of $\frac{1}{4}$, $\frac{3}{8}$, $\frac{1}{2}$, or $\frac{5}{8}$ of a circle; $\frac{1}{2}$ curved are the most commonly used

■ Nutrition

What is the normal daily nitrogen and energy requirement?

Daily nitrogen requirement is 0.2 g kg^{-1} day^{-1} (usually 9 g N day^{-1} for males; 7.5 g N day^{-1} for females). Daily energy requirements are 20–30 kCal kg^{-1} day^{-1} (usually 2500 kcal for males; 2000 kcal for females). Energy requirements are increased in post-operative patients, sepsis, head injury and burns. An energy supply (mixture of carbohydrates and fat) of 30 kCal kg^{-1} day^{-1} is sufficient for most patients. Energy requirements are reduced in unconscious sedated patients on mechanical ventilation. Patients with increased energy requirements will also require increased nitrogen up to 0.4 g kg^{-1} day^{-1}.

Why is it essential to ensure that surgical patients are well nourished?

Malnutrition is associated with increased postoperative morbidity and mortality. Additionally, the reduced immunity increases the risk of postoperative infections.

What are the indications for nutritional support in the surgical patient?

- Malnourished patients: BMI <19; >30% recent weight loss; serum albumin <30 g/l
- Moderate malnutrition: >10% recent weight loss or reduced nutrient intake for >2 weeks preceding surgery
- Impending malnutrition: patients who have a normal nutritional status but are likely to become malnourished if

nutritional support is not provided in the post-operative period, e.g. ventilated patients

How can the nutritional status of a patient be assessed clinically?

- History: dietary intake, recent weight loss
- Examination: reduced muscle strength, peripheral oedema, angular stomatitis, gingivitis, nail abnormalities
- Body mass index (BMI): weight (kg)/height^2 (m^2). Normally 20–25; <19 = malnourishment
- Anthropometric assessment: triceps skin fold thickness, mid arm circumference, hand grip strength
- Bloods: reduced serum albumin or transferrin

What are the different methods of administering nutrition?

- Enteral route: oral supplements; enteral tube feeding (nasogastric, nasojejunal, PEG, PEJ)
- Parenteral route (TPN): routes of administration include: peripheral line (suitable for feeds with <2000 kcal day^{-1} with <14 g N); central line (suitable for feeds with greater energy content and for prolonged feeding)

What are the different types of enteral diets?

- Polymeric diets: indicated for most patients; contains triglyceride and glucose polymers (energy source), whole protein (nitrogen source), electrolytes, trace elements, and vitamins
- Pre-digested diets: indicated in patients with short bowel syndrome or exocrine pancreatic insufficiency; contains long/medium chain triglycerides and long chain glucose polymers (energy source), and free amino acids or oligopeptides (nitrogen source)

- Disease-specific diets: e.g. for patients with respiratory or liver disorders

What are the advantages and disadvantages of enteral nutrition?

Advantages:
- maintains the physiological role of the GIT
- increases GIT blood flow which may prevent the development of sepsis
- no central venous access required
- protects against stress ulceration
- cheaper than TPN

Disadvantages:
- requires a functioning GIT
- problems with feeding tubes: nasal ulceration, sinusitis, tube displacement and blockage, infection
- gastro-oesophageal reflux
- GIT upset: nausea, vomiting, diarrhoea, bloating, abdominal distention

What are the advantages and disadvantages of TPN?

Advantages:
- does not requires a functioning GIT
- all of the nutrition enters the systemic circulation

Disadvantages:
- problems associated with the line: pneumothorax, haemothorax, neurovascular damage, thoracic duct injury, thrombosis, air embolus, thrombophlebitis
- metabolic disturbances: hyponatraemia, hypernatraemia, hypokalaemia, hyperkalaemia, hyperglycaemia, hyperchloraemia, trace element and folate deficiency, linoleic acid deficiency

- hepatic dysfunction
- more expensive than enteral nutrition
- can cause GIT atrophy
- need for regular monitoring of: weight, U&E's, LFTs, Mg^{2+}, Ca^{2+}, PO_4^{2-}, Zn^{2+} and nitrogen balance

■ Obesity and Surgery

Define obesity

Obesity is defined as a body mass index (BMI) of >30; morbid obesity is a BMI >40.

What are the potential problems of surgery in the obese patient?

Pre-operatively:

- patients may have associated medical problems:
  - cardiovascular: left ventricular hypertrophy, cardiomyopathy, systemic and pulmonary hypertension, coronary artery disease, arrhythmias
  - respiratory: reduced lung compliance and functional residual capacity, pulmonary hypertension, chronic hypoxia, hypercapnia and sleep apnoea
  - gastro-intestinal: hiatus hernia and gastro-oesophageal reflux
  - endocrine: diabetes mellitus, hypothyroidism and Cushing's syndrome
- diagnosis of abdominal pain is more difficult
- increased incidence of DVT due to immobility

Operatively:

- anaesthetic difficulties with:
  - intubation and airway maintenance
  - extubation and oxygenation
  - ventilation due to reduced chest wall compliance
  - laryngeal mask airway due to increased risk of aspiration of gastric contents
  - placement of iv lines

- non-invasive blood pressure monitoring
- recovery from some intravenous anaesthetic agents (e.g. thiopentone) may be prolonged
- volatile anaesthetics which predispose to hepatitis especially in obese patients
- positioning difficulties on the operating table:
  - more staff are required for patient transfer
  - table must be strong and wide enough for safe positioning
  - increased incidence of pressure injuries
  - some patients may be unable to lie flat due to respiratory compromise
- surgery can be complicated by technical difficulties because of:
  - limited exposure increasing the likelihood of trauma to associated structures
  - blood loss is greater due to surgery being more technically difficult
  - problems with minimally invasive surgery due to difficulties in gaining access to the peritoneal cavity
  - blood vessels are less well supported and tend to retract when divided therefore, haemorrhage control and subsequent haematoma formation is more likely resulting in increased incidence of wound infection

Post-operatively: obese patients have a higher incidence of:

- respiratory complications including basal lung collapse, atelectasis, hypoxia and infections; ITU or HDU admission may be required
- DVT because intraoperatively the patient's weight exerts a greater pressure on the calf veins and obese patients are often less mobile post surgery
- wound infections and wound dehiscence due to longer incisions, greater wound retraction and the poor blood supply to adipose tissues

- pressure sores
- incisional hernias
- increased analgesic requirements

What specific problems may be encountered in orthopaedic surgery in the obese patient?

Obesity increases the risk of osteoarthritis. Lower limb joint replacements are technically more challenging in obese patients. Furthermore, the excess weight places extra strain on the prosthesis thus increasing the potential for failure. Such patients may require bariatric surgery, i.e. vertical banded gastroplasty to provide weight loss before consideration for joint arthroplasty.

■ Oliguria

Define oliguria and anuria

Oliguria is urine output < 0.5 ml/kg per hour. Anuria is failure to pass any urine.

What are the causes of post-operative oliguria?

- Pre-renal:
  - reduced cardiac output
  - shock (hypovolaemic, cardiogenic, septic)
- Renal:
  - reduced renal perfusion secondary to pre-renal causes
  - acute tubular necrosis, e.g. following nephrotoxic drugs
  - glomerulonephritis
  - acute interstitial nephritis
- Post-renal:
  - benign prostatic hypertrophy
  - blocked catheter
  - ureteric calculus or carcinoma
  - iatrogenic: ureteric ligation

Which commonly used drugs are nephrotoxic?

- Non-steroidal anti-inflammatory drugs, e.g. ibuprofen, diclofenac
- Aminoglycosides, e.g. gentamicin
- ACE inhibitors, e.g. lisinopril
- Thiazide diuretics, e.g. bendroflumethazide

What is the management of oliguria?

- Pre-renal cause:
  - correct hypovolaemia and hypotension by giving fluid challenge. If there is no improvement consider a diuretic

- Renal cause:
  - stop nephrotoxic drugs
  - treat underlying conditions
  - renal replacement therapy
  - nutritional support
  - if no improvement consider a diuretic
- Post-renal cause:
  - if patient not catheterised, insert a catheter
  - bladder washout if catheterised
  - if no improvement perform ultrasound scan to assess for obstructive causes
- Monitor:
  - accurate fluid balance chart

What investigations should be performed in a patient with post-operative oliguria?
- Urine analysis and microscopy
- Serum urea and electrolytes
- Arterial blood gases (assess for acidosis)
- Ultrasound scan to assess for obstructive causes

What are the complications of oliguria?
- Acute renal failure
- Hyperkalaemia

■ Operating Theatre Design

Where should an operating theatre be located within the hospital?
- On the first floor, away from the main hospital traffic
- On the same level and adjacent to ITU and the surgical wards
- Within minimum distance from the A and E and radiology departments

What do you understand by an antiseptic environment within an operating suite?
This consists of four areas:

• Outer (general access zone)	i.e. reception area, general offices
• Clean (limited access zone)	i.e. area between reception bay and theatre suite
• Restricted access zone	i.e. for those properly dressed; anaesthetic room; scrub-up area
• Aseptic zone	Operating area

What is the source of clean air in theatres?
Air is obtained from outside the theatre suite at the roof level and filtered through high efficiency particulate air filters which are capable of filtering microscopic particles with a very high efficiency.

What do the terms turbulent and laminar air flow mean?
In *turbulent (phlenum) flow* there is positive pressure with random airflow. Decreasing pressures from the operating room to the exterior ensure airborne organisms will be carried

out of the operating room. However, there is still the potential for circulation of air within the theatre thereby carrying airborne organisms from the ground level into the operative field. There should be a minimum of 20 air changes per hour to maintain an aerobic count of <35 micro-organisms carrying particles per cubic millimetre. Turbulent flow is necessary to maintain humidity, temperature and air circulation within the operating room.

In *laminar flow* there is positive pressure with parallel airflow. Air is pumped into the operating room through filters and passes out of vents located at the periphery of the operating room. This air does not return back into the operating area. Laminar flow may be vertical or horizontal. Most theatres have 20–40 air changes per hour.

What should the normal temperature be within an operating room? How can heat loss be reduced during surgery?

Normal theatre temperature should be 20–22 °C and is controlled via the ventilation system. This should be increased when operating on neonates, children or the elderly. During prolonged procedures, patients will become hypothermic if the temperature drops below 21 °C. Heat loss can be reduced by using warming blankets and infusion of warm fluids.

What features are important in operating tables?

They should be:
- heavy and stable
- mobile
- comfortable
- adjustable
- radiolucent (thus allowing image intensification to be used)

■ Osteoarthritis I

What are the non-operative methods of treating osteoarthritis (OA)?

- Advice and reassurance regarding the diagnosis
- Modification of activities which aggravate the symptoms
- Weight reduction for lower limb joints
- Walking aids
- Aids to daily living: may help the patient cope with disability, e.g. toilet extenders, safety rails, bath seats
- Shoe raise to overcome shortening associated with hip and knee OA
- Physiotherapy to strengthen muscles around affected joints, increase range of movements and prevent contractures
- Drugs
  - analgesics: to reduce the pain associated with rubbing of raw bone surfaces
  - anti-inflammatories: to reduce synovitis associated with OA
- Intra-articular injections:
  - steroid: to reduce the synovitis associated with OA
  - hyaluronate: increases synovial fluid viscoelasticity and also appears to convey some anti-inflammatory effect

What are the operative options for treating osteoarthritis?

- Debridement and lavage: of osteophytes, loose bodies and articular cartilage debris, which may obstruct joint movement
- Arthrodesis (joint fusion): best suited to osteoarthritis confined to a single joint surrounded by healthy joints. The

joint should be fixed in the most useful functional position for the patient. It will result in a stiff joint and is therefore only useful for small joints of the hand, fingers and toes

- Osteotomy: will correct any deformity and reduce the abnormal load placed across the degenerative joint and will allow remodelling to occur at the osteotomy site. This procedure is associated with significant morbidity, long rehabilitation periods and recurrence of symptoms
- Arthroplasty: creation of a joint which can be:
  - excision arthroplasty, e.g. Girdlestone's procedure, Keller's procedure. Involves excision of both joint surfaces and allows a fibrous union to form between the bone ends. It will create a joint with less movement and stability and is therefore only suitable for non-weight-bearing joints or rarely as a salvage procedure in weight bearing joints
  - interposition arthroplasty: soft tissue, muscle, a liner or spacer can be inserted between the two bone ends to encourage the formation of a pseudoarthrosis. It produces an unstable joint and results are similar to excision arthroplasty
  - hemiarthroplasty, e.g. Austin Moore hip hemiarthroplasty; involves excision and replacement of one joint surface only. The disadvantage is that the prosthetic material may wear away the opposite surface
  - unicompartmental arthroplasty, e.g. Oxford uni-compartmental knee replacement; involves excision and replacement of one compartment of both joint surfaces
  - total replacement arthroplasty, e.g. total hip replacement. Excision and replacement of both joint surfaces produces an anatomically more stable joint

■ Osteoarthritis II: Hip

What are the operative options for osteoarthritis of the hip?

- Upper femoral osteotomy: can be varus or valgus osteotomy; the principle is to realign the weight-bearing surface of the hip joint. Mainly suitable for younger patients with femoral head collapse and with a reasonable range of movements
- Arthrodesis: rarely performed in modern times; occasionally appropriate for severe osteoarthritis secondary to trauma in young patients
- Hip resurfacing: bone conserving procedure in which the head of the femur is reshaped and resurfaced, rather than being removed. Since both parts of the bearing surfaces are made of metal, the resurfacing hip system is intended to last much longer and therefore is more suitable for higher demand patients
- Total hip replacement: both the acetabular and femoral components are replaced:
  - acetabular component: usually made of high density polyethylene which is biocompatible and has a low rate of wear; ceramic acetabular components have improved surface properties but are expensive and have a tendency to brittle failure; metal cups are rarely used due to high rates of loosening and wear
  - femoral component: usually made of stainless steel, titanium or cobalt chrome alloy, which are corrosion resistant
  - cemented implants: polymethylmethacrylate (cement) is used to secure prosthetic components in situ. Addition of

antibiotics to the cement may reduce the incidence of infection

- uncemented implants: porous-coated components which are anchored by interference fit initially and then rely on bone ingrowth between the pores for stability; hydroxyapatite coating to the pores increases bony ingrowth and strength of fixation. Uncemented implants reduce the problem of mechanical loosening encountered with cemented implants which is a significant problem especially in the younger patient

What are the advantages of hip resurfacing?

- Femoral head and canal are preserved
- Larger size of implant 'ball' reduces the incidence of dislocation
- Stress is transferred in a natural way along the femoral canal and through the head and neck of the femur. With standard total hip replacements, bone has to respond and reform to less natural stress loading, resulting in thigh pain
- Use of metal rather than plastic reduces the risk of bone loss, early loosening and has a low wear rate with increased implant longevity

■ Osteoarthritis III: Knee

What are the operative options for osteoarthritis of the knee?

- Arthroscopic debridement: indicated in patients with mild degenerative joint disease with mechanical symptoms and recurrent persistent effusions. Arthroscopy will also allow a thorough inspection of the joint so a firm prognosis can be offered
- Osteotomy: reserved for young high-demand patients because of concerns about the durability of total knee replacement in these patients
  - proximal tibial valgus osteotomy: can be considered in patients with medial tibio-femoral compartment disease with a healthy lateral compartment, stable collateral ligaments, and a correctable varus deformity
  - distal femoral varus osteotomy: mainly used in patients with lateral tibio-femoral compartment disease, stable collateral ligaments, and a correctable valgus deformity
- Arthrodesis: rarely performed and is reserved for patients with chronic sepsis; younger patients with tricompartmental disease (e.g. following trauma) who require stability and durability; and patients with deficient extensor mechanisms
- Unicompartmental knee replacement: can be used in low-demand patients with unicompartmental disease
- Total knee replacement: these can be of three general types:
  - unconstrained prostheses: metal and plastic components are secured separately to the tibial and femoral surfaces of each component. Only used in stable joints with intact ligaments as the components simply resurface the joint and do not contribute to the stability of the joint

- semi-constrained prostheses: used for patients with more moderate degenerative disease. The whole of both joint surfaces and the patella are replaced and contribute to the stability of the joint
- fully constrained (hinged) prostheses: mechanically links the two parts of the prostheses and is reserved for an unstable joint with a poor bone stock

■ Osteomyelitis

Define osteomyelitis

It is infection of bone leading to inflammatory destruction of bone, bone necrosis and new bone formation. It can be acute, sub-acute or chronic.

Which pathogens usually cause osteomyelitis?

- Neonates: Streptococci (group B), *S. aureus*, gram-negative bacteria
- Age 3–15: *S. aureus*, Streptococci (group A)
- Adults: *S. aureus*

Describe the pathogenesis of acute osteomyelitis

- Dental sepsis, trivial wounds or scratches cause bacteraemia
- Convoluted arrangement of metaphyseal blood vessels act as functional 'end-arterioles' trapping bacteria in this region, which initiate an inflammatory response
- Stage 1: infection usually begins in medulla of long bones
- Stage 2: pus tracks through cortex to form a subperiosteal abscess, which causes periosteal stripping and new bone formation
- Stage 3: abscess forms in soft tissues
- New bone formed (involucrum) envelopes the surrounding necrotic area
- Avascular cortical bone can separate from the rest of bone to create holes (cloacae) and give rise to large islands of dead bone in sea of pus or granulation tissue (sequestra)

What are the symptoms of acute osteomyelitis?
- Rapid onset bone pain and tenderness in affected areas, often metaphysis of long bones
- Fevers, rigors and malaise, especially in children
- Erythema and swelling may develop quickly if treatment is not commenced. The child with acute osteomyelitis may refuse to use the affected limb
- There may be no localising signs in young infants
- The unwell child with bone tenderness has osteomyelitis until proven otherwise

What investigations may be useful in diagnosing acute osteomyelitis?
- Bloods:
  - elevated WCC, CRP, ESR
  - blood cultures – positive in 50%
- X-ray: changes lag behind clinical picture and may be normal in the early stages
  - soft tissue swelling, periosteal reaction, new bone formation, lytic lesions
- USS: can identify subperiosteal fluid which can be aspirated for further analysis
- Bone scan – 'hot spot' may be in affected area
- MRI

What is the management of acute osteomyelitis?
This involves:
- antibiotics
- surgical drainage of pus ± debridement

Describe chronic osteomyelitis
It is normally the consequence of late diagnosis or inadequate treatment of acute osteomyelitis. There are four types: medullary, superficial, localised and diffuse. There is usually a

history of previous infection, gradual onset bone pain especially on weight-bearing. Examination may reveal a source of infection i.e. overlying chronic ulceration, septicaemia or a discharge from an overlying sinus. Investigations are as for acute osteomyelitis. MRI may be useful in the assessment for the extent of bony involvement.

What is the management of chronic osteomyelitis?
- Occasional flares settle with antibiotics
- Aims of surgical treatment are:
  - adequate debridement of pus and all dead bone
  - stabilisation of skeleton with an external fixator
  - plastic surgery to restore soft tissue cover
  - reconstitution of bony continuity with autologous cancellous bone graft or vascularised bone graft

What are the complications of osteomyelitis?
- Septicaemia
- Recurrence
- Pathological fractures
- Skin problems, e.g. malignant change at sites of sinuses
- Amyloidosis
- Growth disturbance in children

Describe subacute osteomyelitis
It is a condition that is becoming increasingly common. The spine is most commonly affected with infection in vertebral end plates or discs in 10–20-year olds. The pelvis can also be affected (osteitis pubis). It is usually caused by *S. aureus* infection. Symptoms include bone pain with no systemic signs of infection. MRI may be useful to aid diagnosis. Treatment options include antibiotics and surgical clearance of the lesion.

■ Paediatric Surgery

Define the terms premature, neonate, infant and child

Premature: born before 37 weeks of gestational age

Neonate: a newborn up to a month of age; in a premature baby the word neonate describes a baby up to 44 weeks post-conceptual age

Infant: age 1 month to 1 year

Child: age 1 year to 16 years

Why is the management of a child's airway different from that of an adult?

In children the:

- head is large and the neck short which predispose to flexion injuries
- large tongue and adenoids can obscure the view during laryngoscopy
- larynx lies at the level of C2/3 compared with at C5/6 in adults
- trachea is short and thus can be compressed with over-extension of the neck
- tubes used should be uncuffed to avoid the cuff irritating the cricoid lining

How can the size of an oral endotracheal tube be estimated from the child's age?

In children over 1 year of age the:

- length of the tube (cm) is [age (in years)/2] + 2
- internal diameter (mm) is [age (in years)/4] + 4

List the sites for vascular access in neonates and infants

- Scalp
- Internal jugular vein
- Cubital fossa
- Dorsum of hand
- Femoral vein
- Tibial metaphysis
- Long saphenous vein
- Dorsum of foot

How is fluid requirement calculated in children?

• First 10 kg of weight	4 ml/kg
• Next 10 kg of weight	2 ml/kg
• Weight > 20 kg	1 ml/kg

What is the estimated blood volume in children?

• Neonate (preterm)	100 ml/kg
• Neonate (term)	90 ml/kg
• Infants	80 ml/kg
• Child	70 ml/kg

Why is it important to maintain haemostasis in neonates undergoing surgery?

At birth the average blood volume is 300 ml and loss of only 30 ml (10%) will result in circulatory failure! Neonates are not able to tolerate a fall in circulating volume because they are not able to raise their stroke volume in response and their haemostatic mechanisms are not well developed. In addition, the immaturity of the neonatal hepatic system means that there is inadequate production of clotting factors, which predisposes to bleeding.

Why do neonates develop hypothermia faster than older children or adults?

This is because:
- they have a larger surface to weight ratio
- they have less subcutaneous fat
- premature neonates may have less brown fat which is a heat source
- they cannot shiver normally
- their central thermoregulation centre is immature
- they have poor voluntary thermoregulation

What measures should be undertaken to prevent hypothermia in neonates undergoing surgery?

- Minimise the time they are kept uncovered
- Lie the neonate on a warming blanket and wrap the extremities or use a warm air delivery system
- Increase the operating theatre temperature
- Use of warm intravenous fluids
- Use of warm swabs
- Use of warm fluids to irrigate body cavities

Why are anaesthetists concerned about colds in paediatric patients before surgery?

Upper respiratory tract infection (URTI) is the most common illness in children under 5 years of age. A child with URTI has an increased incidence of:
- laryngospasm during induction of anaesthesia
- bronchospasm
- coughing which can cause regurgitation and aspiration
- reduced oxygen saturation due to above factors, atelectasis and reduced FRC

When should elective surgery be cancelled in children with respiratory tract infections?

- Patients with a lower respiratory tract infection
- Patients < 1 year old with URTI
- Clinical signs of systemic illness
- Patients that may require oral endotracheal intubation

In cases of URTI, surgery should be postponed for 1–2 weeks after cessation of symptoms. For lower respiratory infections, surgery should be delayed for at least 4–6 weeks after cessation of symptoms.

How long should the nil by mouth (NBM) period last?

- Neonates and infants <6 months of age can continue to have formula or breast milk up to 6 h before surgery, followed by clear fluids until 3 h before surgery
- Older infants and children should refrain from milk for 6 h before surgery but can have clear fluids until 3 h before surgery

Is there an increased anaesthetic risk in children compared with adults?

Yes. The incidence of cardiac arrest under anaesthesia is about three times higher for the paediatric patient compared with an adult. The enhanced anaesthetic risk is due to:

- difficulty with intubation and maintenance of airway due to reasons described above
- children having frequent URTIs which predisposes their airways to remain reactive for up to 7 weeks following the onset of symptoms
- increased risk of malignant hyperthermia
- congenital abnormalities of major organs
- anaphylaxis occurring in patients with undiagnosed latex allergy

Which group of children require pre-operative clearance of their cervical spine prior to surgery?

Patients with:

- arthritis: especially juvenile rheumatoid arthritis
- bone dysplasias: can lead to odontoid malformation
- chromosomal anomalies especially Down's syndrome
- congenital scoliosis

List commonly used analgesics in the paediatric patient

• Paracetamol	10–15 mg/kg
• Ibuprofen	5 mg/kg
• Diclofenac	1 mg/kg (usually given rectally)
• Morphine	0.1–0.2 mg/kg (<1 yr); 0.2–0.4 mg/kg (>1 yr)

- Local anaesthetics: applied topically but not on broken skin
  - EMLA® (2.5% lignocaine and 2.5% prilocaine): onset of effect at 45 mins and duration of action of 60 min
  - Ametop® (4% amethocaine): onset of effect at 45 min and duration of action of about 4 hours

■ Pain

Define pain
An unpleasant sensory and/or emotional experience associated with actual or potential tissue damage.

What are the principles of post-operative pain management?
- Pre-operative:
  - pre-emptive analgesia, e.g. NSAIDs or nerve blocks
  - patient education
- Intra-operative:
  - use of opioid analgesics
  - regional nerve blocks
  - wound infiltration with local anaesthetics
- Post-operative:
  - pharmacological therapy
  - regional anaesthetic blocks
  - alternative methods

How can post-operative pain be assessed?
- Subjectively
- Objectively:
  - verbal numerical scale
  - visual analogue scale

What are the systemic effects of post-operative pain?
- Cardiovascular:
  - enhanced myocardial O_2 demand
  - myocardial ischaemia

- increased sympathetic stimulation ⇒ increased cardiac output ⇒ reduced renal and splanchnic perfusion
- Respiratory:
  - decrease cough ⇒ sputum retention ⇒ chest infection
  - hypoxia
- Gastrointestinal:
  - reduced G.I. motility ⇒ constipation
  - ileus
- Genitourinary:
  - urinary retention
- Metabolic:
  - hyperglycaemia
  - hypernatraemia
- Psychological:
  - stress
  - depression
- General:
  - increase hospital in-stay

List some commonly used analgesics in the post-operative period

Drug	Mode of action	Route	Adverse effects
Paracetamol	Modulates PGE2 in the central nervous system	po, pr, iv	Rare: unless in overdose causes liver failure
NSAIDs (e.g. ibuprofen, diclofenac)	inhibits cyclo-oxygenase	po, pr, iv, im	gastritis, peptic ulceration, renal failure, bronchospasm in asthmatics, bleeding

Drug	Mode of action	Route	Adverse effects
Weak opiates (e.g. codeine phosphate)	Act on Mu 1 receptors in the central nervous system	po, sc, iv, im, pca	Sedation, CNS depression, respiratory depression, nausea, vomiting, itching, constipation
Strong opiates (e.g. pethidine, morphine, fentanyl)		Epidural, spinal	

How are local anaesthetics used in post-operative pain relief?

They can be:

- infiltrated directly into the surgical wound
- used in regional blocks
- used in epidurals

What are the alternative methods of pain relief?

- Good patient education
- Relaxation techniques
- Acupuncture
- Trans-cutaneous electrical nerve stimulation (TENS)

■ Perioperative Monitoring

What parameters must be monitored in all anaesthetised patients?
- Respiratory
  - inspired O_2 (Fi O_2)
  - pulse oximetry
  - end-tidal CO_2
- Cardiovascular
  - heart rate
  - blood pressure
  - ECG
  - invasive blood pressure
    monitoring   (usually only in major surgery)
  - central venous pressure   (usually only in major surgery)
- Temperature

What effects do general anaesthetics have on the core body temperature?
They cause hypothermia due to their vasodilatory effects. Radiation of body heat and evaporation from open body cavities along with administration of cold intravenous fluids reduce the temperature further. Heat loss can be minimised by using warming blankets (bear huggers), infusing warm fluids and using warm fluids to irrigate body cavities.

List the possible causes of failure to spontaneously breathe after general anaesthesia
- Airway difficulties due to:
  - obstruction
- Breathing difficulties due to:

- central depression caused by anaesthetic agents or opiates
- hypoxia
- hypercarbia
- pneumothorax
- Circulatory failure

Peripheral Vascular Disease

What are the risk factors for the development of peripheral vascular disease?
- Increasing age
- Male sex
- Smoking
- Hypertension
- Hyperlipidaemia
- Diabetes mellitus
- Family history

What are the clinical features of chronic lower limb ischaemia?
Symptoms:
- intermittent claudication: site of arterial occlusion determines the muscle group affected, e.g. aorto-iliac disease causes thigh and buttock pain; femoro-popliteal disease results in thigh and calf pain; distal disease causes calf and foot pain
- rest pain: pain worse at night and exacerbated on elevation of foot; improved with hanging the foot over the side of the bed; pain worse at night

Signs:
- cold peripheries
- weak or absent pulses
- increased capillary refill time
- trophic changes
- gangrene
- arterial ulcers
- venous guttering

Define critical limb ischaemia

European Consensus Document on Critical Limb Ischaemia defined this as:

- persistently recurring rest pain requiring analgesia for >2 weeks
- ulceration or gangrene of the foot or toes with an ankle pressure <50 mmHg
- toe systolic pressure < 30 mmHg
- transcutaneous oxygen pressure of the ischaemic area ($tcPO_2$) < 10 mmHg and which does not increase with inhalation of oxygen
- absence of arterial pulsation in big toe (measured with strain gauge or photoplethysmography after vasodilatation)
- marked structural or functional change of skin capillaries in the affected area

Which investigations may be useful in the assessment of chronic lower limb ischaemia?

General investigations:
- Bloods:
  - FBC, CRP, ESR: underlying haematological or inflammatory cause
  - U and Es: impaired renal function due to renovascular disease
  - cholesterol and glucose
  - clotting screen: prior to angioplasty or surgery
  - ECG/ exercise ECG: underlying cardiac disease
  - CXR: cardiomegaly
  - thallium scan/echocardiogram: patients with suspected or established cardiac disease prior to surgery

Specific investigations:
- Ankle–brachial pressure index: normally >1.0; claudication occurs at 0.4–0.7 and critical ischaemia at 0.1–0.4

- Resting and post-exercise doppler pressures: differentiates pain on walking caused by arterial insufficiency from pain on walking due to other causes
- Duplex ultrasound: advantages include non-invasive procedure, inexpensive and reproducible; disadvantages are: it is operator-dependent and produces poor quality images
- Angiography: can be intravenous digital subtraction (IVDSA) or intra-arterial digital subtraction (IADSA). Performed under local anaesthetic. Advantages of IADSA over IVDSA are: a smaller contrast load is required, produces images with good resolution and allows intervention if required. Disadvantages are: it is not repeatable and requires an arterial puncture. Complications include: anaphylactic or toxic reaction to the contrast, infection, haematoma, arterial spasm, false aneurysm, AV fistula, acute thrombosis and distal embolisation.
- CT angiography: requires intravenous contrast
- Magnetic resonance angiography: no contrast required

What are the non-surgical treatment options for chronic lower limb ischaemia?

- Modify risk factors
  - stop smoking
  - reduce weight
  - treat and control hyperlipidaemia, diabetes mellitus, and hypertension
- Regular exercise to allow collateral circulation to develop
- Drug therapy
  - Aspirin (75–300 mg)
  - Naftidrofuryl and petoxifylline: useful in intermittent claudication
  - Prostanoids: for critical limb ischaemia
  - Iloprost® : improves rest pain and ulcer healing

Peripheral Vascular Disease

- Lumbar sympathectomy: may relieve mild rest pain and aid superficial ulcer healing; minimal benefit for intermittent claudication
- Epidural spinal cord stimulation: produces paraesthesia in the lower limbs and may be useful in pain control in healing of small ulcers

What are the indications for intervention in peripheral vascular disease?
- Critical limb ischaemia
- Disabling claudication

What are the options?
- Percutaneous transluminal angioplasty ± stenting: optimal results observed with short segment stenoses <2 cm long and for proximal stenoses
- Endarterectomy
- Bypass surgery
- Amputation: for patients with unreconstructable peripheral vascular disease

What are the principles of arterial reconstructive surgery?
- Optimisation of the patient's co-existing conditions with relevant investigations being performed
- Arteriography to determine the exact site of obstruction, length of obstruction and distal run-off, i.e. patient vessels distal to the occlusion
- Types of graft can be:
  - autografts: long sapphenous vein (valves destroyed or vein reversed); internal mammary artery
  - allografts: Dacron® coated umbilical vein
  - synthetic grafts: Dacron®, woven graft or polyfluorotetraethylene (PTFE)

- Choice of graft material determined by site of occlusion, length of occlusion, availability of suitable vein graft and long-term patency rates (higher for vein than PTFE)
- For aorto-iliac disease, a trouser or 'Y' prosthetic graft often used; for femoro-popliteal disease, vein graft used
- Reasons for graft failure: immediately due to technical failure; early failure due to intimal hyperplasia at distal anastomosis and late failure most often due to progression of distal disease
- Complications of surgery:
  - general: acute MI, CVA, renal failure
  - local: haemorrhage, thrombosis, embolism, infection, pseudoaneurysm formation

What are the causes of acute lower limb ischaemia?
- Embolus (left atrium in patients with AF; mural thrombus after a recent MI; prosthetic heart valves)
- Acute thrombosis
- Vasospastic disorders, e.g. Raynaud's phenomenon, cryoglobulinaemia

How can acute occlusion by thrombosis and embolus be differentiated?
Patients with a thrombus may have evidence of chronic arterial disease and abnormal pulses noted in the contralateral limb. In contrast, patients presenting with an embolus may have an obvious cardiac source with no history of claudication and normal pulses are noted in the contralateral limb.

What are the clinical features of acute lower limb ischaemia?
- Pain
- Pallor
- Paraesthesia

- Paralysis
- Pulselessness
- Perishingly cold

What is the management of acute lower limb ischaemia?

- Oxygenation, fluid resuscitation and adequate analgesia
- Treat underlying cause, e.g. atrial fibrillation
- Intravenous heparin
- Aspirin
- Embolic disease: embolectomy or intra-arterial thrombolysis
- Thrombotic disease: intra-arterial thrombolysis, angioplasty or reconstructive surgery
- Amputation if limb not viable

Physiological Response to Surgery

What is the physiological response to surgery?

It is a systemic reaction following surgery, which encompasses a wide range of sympathetic, endocrinal, immunological and haematological effects. The extent of response is proportional to severity of insult caused by surgery.

Describe the endocrine response following surgery

Endocrine gland	Hormone	Changes in secretion	Systemic effect
Anterior pituitary	ACTH Growth hormone	↑ ↑	Stimulates cortisol secretion from the adrenal cortex, simulates lipolysis
Posterior pituitary	ADH	↑	Increases water resorption and produces vasoconstriction
Adrenal cortex	Aldosterone Cortisol	↑ ↑	Increases sodium resorption, protein catabolism, lipolysis, glycogenolysis, gluconeogenesis
Pancreas	Insulin Glucagon	↓ ↑	Hyperglycaemia
Thyroid	Thyroxine, T3	↓	Reason for the changes remain unclear

What are the metabolic sequelae of the endocrine response?

- Carbohydrate metabolism: blood glucose concentrations increase after surgery. Hyperglycaemia is caused by increased hepatic glycogenolysis and gluconeogenesis, decreased peripheral glucose use, increased glucose production and relative lack of insulin together with peripheral insulin resistance
- Protein catabolism: predominantly, skeletal muscle is broken down, but some visceral muscle protein is also catabolised to release amino acids which may be further catabolised for energy or used in the liver to form new proteins, particularly acute-phase proteins. Protein catabolism results in marked weight loss and muscle wasting in patients after major surgery
- Fat metabolism: fat stored as triglyceride is converted by lipolysis to glycerol and fatty acids
- Water and electrolyte metabolism: water and sodium is retained to maintain fluid volume and cardiovascular homeostasis

Describe the neuronal response following surgery

Hypothalamic activation of the sympathetic autonomic nervous system results in increased secretion of catecholamines from the adrenal medulla and release of noradrenaline from pre-synaptic nerve terminals. The increased sympathetic activity results in:

- cardiovascular effects: tachycardia, hypertension, increased myocardial contractility, and blood being diverted from skin and visceral organs to the site of surgical insult
- respiratory effects: bronchodilation
- gastro-intestinal effects: reduced motility

- metabolic effects: reduced insulin production, increased glucagon production and increased glycogenolysis causing hyperglycaemia

What is the role of the immune system in surgical trauma?

Surgical insult stimulates cytokine release mainly TNF-α, IL-1, IL-2, IL-6, interferon and prostaglandins, which are important in regulating the inflammatory response. Hyper-stimulation of cytokine production and its subsequent release into the systemic circulation can cause systemic inflammatory response syndrome (SIRS).

Cytokines also stimulate the production of acute phase proteins such as C-reactive protein (CRP), fibrinogen, complement C3 and α_2-macroglobulin.

What is the role of the vascular endothelium in surgical trauma?

It produces:
- nitric oxide and prostaglandins, which cause vasodilatation
- platelet activating factor, which enhances the cytokine response

Does the mode of anaesthesia influence the systemic response to surgery?

Yes. Although anaesthesia has little effect on the cytokine response to surgery (because it cannot influence tissue trauma), the use of regional anaesthesia with local anaesthetic agents or in combination with opioids has been shown to reduce the stress response to surgery in the pelvis and the lower limbs but not with upper abdominal or thoracic surgery. Furthermore, they can also influence post-operative outcome by beneficial effects on organ function.

Does minimally invasive surgery reduce the systemic response to surgery?

No. Although minimally invasive surgery causes less IL-6 and CRP production compared with conventional surgery, the metabolic response is not reduced in minimally invasive surgery. The overall effect is that there is no change in the physiological response by reducing surgical trauma.

■ Positioning of Patients

What problems are encountered during positioning of surgical patients?

Supine position:

- ↑ CVP ⇒ ↑ C.O. (this in turn causes ↓ heart rate)
- ventilation and perfusion becomes more uniform

Trendeleburgh position:

- ↑ CVP ⇒ ↑ C.O. (this in turn causes ↓ heart rate)
- venous congestion and oedema in the head and neck
- ↑ pressure from abdominal contents on to the diaphragm will reduce the lung's functional residual capacity

Lithotomy position:

- sacro-iliac joint strain: due to excessive flexion of the hips and knees
- hip dislocation: if lithotomy poles slip
- compartment syndrome: due to pressure on calf muscles by stirrups
- injury to nerves: sciatic, common peroneal, tibial, obturator, femoral

What are the causes of nerve injuries in the anaesthetised patient?

- Poor positioning of patients
- Ischaemia secondary to:
  - tourniquets
  - hypotension
- During administration of regional anaesthesia, e.g. femoral nerve injury during nerve blockade

What nerve injuries are encountered during positioning of patients? How can they be prevented?

Nerve	Mechanism of injury	Prevention
Ulnar (most common)	Compression at the elbow between the medial epicondyle and the edge of operating table in a pronated arm	Arms positioned in supination
Radial	• compression between humeral shaft and edge of operating table or arm board • tourniquet injury	• prevent arm hanging freely over table edge • adequate padding of tourniquets
Brachial plexus	Stretched during arm movements especially when shoulder abducted >90°	Avoid excessive abduction; avoid arm falling off side of table
Common peroneal	Compression between fibular neck and edge of operating table, especially in the lithotomy or Lloyd Davis positions	Adequate padding of lithotomy poles
Sciatic	Direct compression during prolonged surgery especially in emaciated patients	Adequate padding at the sciatic exit point
Pudendal	Compression against ischial tuberosity by post on traction table	Adequate padding of posts; reduced surgery time
Saphenous	Compression against medial tibial condyle by lithotomy poles	Adequate padding of poles
Supra-orbital	Compression by tracheal tube connectors in the prone position	Adequate positioning of tracheal tube connectors

What other injuries can occur in anaesthetised patients?

- Skin injuries:
  - directly from sticky drapes, ECG electrodes or self adhesive tapes
  - indirectly from diathermy burns or allergies to skin preparation fluids
  - due to ischaemia from prolonged pressure
- Corneal abrasions: prevented by taping the eyelids closed
- Damage to teeth, nasal and oral cavities as a result of trauma during intubation
- Neck injuries and dislocations during moving and positioning of patients
- Compartment syndrome:
  - from use of tourniquets
  - from prolonged direct compression causing increased compartmental pressures
  - from prolonged hypotension especially in the Lloyd–Davies position

Post-operative Care

What are the different levels of post-operative care?

- Recovery room: where it should be ensured that the patient is:
  - transferred from theatre under the supervision of an anaesthetist
  - nursed one-to-one with regular clinical observations
  - maintaining their airway until consciousness returns
  - breathing adequately
  - cardiovascularly stable
  - comfortable
  - given adequate analgesia
- High Dependency Unit (HDU): where nursing staff:
  - to patient ratio is 1 : 3–4
  - are trained to monitor arterial pressure and CVP lines
  - are able to maintain pain relief techniques, e.g. epidurals
- Intensive Care Unit (ICU): where patients:
  - to nursing staff ratio is 1:1
  - are provided with cardiovascular and/or respiratory support
  - are provided with renal support, e.g. dialysis, haemofiltration
- General wards
- Day care wards

Describe the characteristics that a recovery room should possess

It should be:

- close to the operating theatre
- be open plan and well lit

- well equipped with monitoring facilities
- run by appropriately trained staff
- separate areas for adults and children

What are the common problems encountered in the recovery room?

- Respiratory:
  - airway obstruction secondary to: residual effects of anaesthesia or muscle relaxants reducing the tone of oropharangeal muscles; laryngospasm; blood or foreign bodies within the oral cavity or oedema of the laryngopharynx
  - hypoxaemia secondary to: atelectasis, bronchospasm, pneumothorax, pulmonary embolism, pneumonia, pulmonary oedema or shivering
  - hypoventilation secondary to: drugs (anaesthetic agents, opiates, benzodiazepines or neuromuscular blockade), intraoperative positive pressure ventilation, hypothermia or pre-existing respiratory disease
- Cardiovascular:
  - hypotension secondary to: hypovolaemia (inadequate replacement of fluids) and vasodilatation (residual effects of anaesthetic agents)
  - hypertension secondary to: pain, bladder distension, hypercapnia or hypoxia
  - arrhythmias secondary to: co-existing cardiac disease, pain or electrolyte imbalances
- Central nervous system (CNS):
  - pain: if untreated can result in tachycardia, hypertension, increased myocardial oxygen demand, and atelectasis
  - nausea and vomiting: particularly associated with ENT, gynaecological and ophthalmic surgery
- Thermoregulation:

- hypothermia secondary to: residual vasodilatory effects of general anaesthetics, radiation of body heat or administration of cold intravenous fluids
- hyperthermia secondary to: sepsis, over-active re-warming or blood transfusion reactions

■ Post-operative Complications

List the common complications encountered in the post-operative period

Respiratory:

- Atelectasis: a common cause of post-operative pyrexia. Incidence can be minimised with pre-operative patient education, early mobilisation and encouragement to cough. Treatment consists of lung expansion and clearing of secretions
- Pneumonia: often caused by aspiration of pathogens from the oropharynx. Increased incidence in ventilated patients. Common organism includes *Pseudomonas aeruginosa, Enterobacter, Staph. aureus, Haemophilus influenzae* and anaerobes. Treatment consists of adequate oxygenation, clearance of any secretions and commencement of appropriate antibiotics
- Pulmonary oedema: treatment involves correcting the underlying cause, use of diuretics and careful monitoring of fluid balance
- Aspiration pneumonitis: chemical pneumonitis occurs as a result of aspiration of gastric contents. Most commonly seen in apical segments of right lower lobe. It can result in a secondary bacterial infection usually with gram-negative and anaerobic organisms
- Pulmonary embolism: prevention methods as for DVT prophylaxis. Treatment includes anticoagulation, thrombolysis, embolectomy or insertion of caval filters
- Pleural effusion: common after abdominal surgery. Occasionally due to subphrenic abscess

Cardiac:

- Arrhythmias: most common rhythm is atrial fibrillation which, if associated with haemodynamic instability, requires prompt treatment. Sinus tachycardia is most commonly caused by pain, hypovolaemia or hypotension. Sinus bradycardia may be due to residual effects of anaesthetic agents, hypoxaemia or myocardial infarction
- Hypertension: usually due to uncontrolled pain, pre-existing hypertension, hypoxaemia, hypercapnia or effects of positive inotropic drugs
- Hypotension: usually due to residual effects of anaesthetic agents or opioids, hypovolaemia, perioperative MI or sepsis
- Myocardial infarction
- Cardiac failure: common causes include fluid overload, MI and arrhythmias

Urinary tract:

- Infection: mainly due to bacterial colonisation of catheters. Common pathogens include *E. coli, Proteus mirabilis, Pseudomonas aeruginosa* and *Enterococcus*. Risk of catheter-related infection is higher in the elderly, in those with urological diseases and patients who have had an indwelling catheter for > 2 weeks
- Retention: common after major surgery or operations under spinal/epidural anaesthesia

Pyrexia: (discussed under pyrexia)

Wound:

- Infection: usually apparent 3–7 days after surgery and may be associated with surrounding cellulites. Superficial infections can be treated with appropriate antibiotics but deeper infections require formal exploration and washout
- Haematoma: predispose to wound infections and may require formal exploration and washout
- Dehiscence: (discussed under wound healing)

Renal failure: (discussed under oliguria)

Gastrointestinal:

- Paralytic ileus (discussed under small bowel obstruction)
- Pseudo-obstruction (discussed under large bowel obstruction)

Hepatobiliary:

- Hepatic dysfunction: common causes include blood transfusion, haemolytic disorders, pre-existing hepatic disease, viral hepatitis, sepsis, hypotension, hypoxaemia, drug-induced hepatitis (especially halothane), pancreatitis and common bile duct injury
- Acalculous cholecystitis: due to bile stasis and thrombosis of blood vessels within the gall bladder

Confusion: causes include

- Hypoxia: respiratory disease, cardiac failure, arrhythmia
- Infection: wound, chest, urinary, intracranial, extracranial
- Drugs: opioids
- Alcohol withdrawal
- Metabolic disturbance
- Endocrine: hypothyroidism, hyperthyroidism
- Degenerative: acute confusional state on a background of dementia

Nausea and vomiting:

- Usually due to the effects of general anaesthetics and opioids. Pre-emptive antiemetics (cyclizine and metoclopramide) reduce the incidence of post-operative nausea and vomiting

Pre-admission Clinics

What are the advantages of a pre-admission clinic?
- Allows thorough assessment of patients prior to surgery
- Any relevant investigations can be ordered at the time of assessment and any abnormalities corrected prior to admission thus reducing cancellation of operations on the day of surgery
- Any potential post-operative problems can be anticipated and planned for, i.e. the need for an intensive care bed post-surgery
- Any potential anaesthetic problems can be discussed with the anaesthetist prior to surgery
- Patients can be given more information about their proposed surgery and consent can be obtained at the same time
- Permits a rapport to be established with the patient
- Patients can meet allied health care professionals who may be involved with their post-operative care, e.g. specialised nurses, occupational therapists, pharmacists and physiotherapists

What are the disadvantages of a pre-admission clinic?
- Illnesses can arise in the interim period between pre-admission clinic and admission to the ward and therefore patients will need to be reviewed again on admission
- Assessment of patients and investigations will need to be repeated if there is postponement of surgery for more than 4 weeks after attendance to the pre-admission clinic

- Pre-admission clinics are often run by specialist nurses or junior doctors who may not be able to answer all the patient's questions regarding the proposed surgery

How long before the surgery should pre-admission clinics be held?

Not more than 4 weeks prior to surgery.

Who should run pre-admission clinics?

Ideally, the anaesthetist who will be managing the patient on the day of surgery. However, in reality they are often run by the most junior members of the surgical team.

■ Pregnancy

Why should surgeons know something about pregnancy and its complications?

- In the differential diagnosis of abdominal pain:
  - pre-eclampsia
  - uterine rupture
  - uterine torsion
  - pyelonephritis
  - placental abruption
  - HELLP syndrome
  - rectus sheath haematoma
  - acute fatty liver of pregnancy
- Some surgical diseases are more common in pregnancy:
  - acute cholecystitis
  - acute appendicitis

Describe appendicitis in pregnancy

Incidence is 1 in 1000 pregnancies. It is associated with a high incidence of foetal morbidity and mortality especially in the first and second trimesters. Foetal mortality is 5–10% in simple appendicitis and up to 30% when there is a perforation. During pregnancy, the appendix migrates upwards, outwards and posteriorly and thereby the pain of appendicitis is less well localised (often paraumbilical or subcostal) and tenderness, guarding and rebound tenderness are often absent, thus making the diagnosis more difficult. Abdominal ultrasound may be useful if diagnosis is in doubt. Appendicectomy or laparotomy is required.

Describe acute cholecystitis in pregnancy

Incidence is 1–5 per 10 000 pregnancies. In pregnancy, biliary stasis is common and the bile is more concentrated in cholesterol thereby encouraging gallstone formation. Symptoms are similar to the non-pregnant with right upper quadrant or epigastric pain, nausea and vomiting. Ultrasound will confirm the diagnosis. Surgery should be delayed until the baby is delivered or until the foetus is mature enough to withstand delivery (second trimester).

What are the principles of surgery in the pregnant patient?

Pre-operative:
- involve the obstetrician early
- consider pre-eclampsia: routinely monitor blood pressure and perform urinalysis to detect proteinuria
- prophylactic anticoagulation may be required due to increased incidence of thrombosis in pregnancy
- be aware of anaesthetic difficulties, e.g.
  - hypoxaemia due to reduced functional residual capacity as a result of the uterus displacing the diaphragm upwards
  - aspiration of gastric contents at induction due to increased incidence of gastro-oesophageal reflux
- delay non-urgent surgery until the second trimester

Operative:
- position with a left tilt of at least 30° to prevent aorto-caval compression and supine hypotension syndrome

Post-operative:
- care should be taken when prescribing drugs as they may cross the placenta
- prophylactic anticoagulation may be required due to increased incidence of thrombotic events

What is the risk of miscarriage in the first trimester due to surgery and anaesthesia?

It is between 5 and 8%. Risk of onset of premature labour is similar.

■ Pre-medication

What is pre-medication?

It is the administration of any drug prior to surgery. This can be one of the patient's normal prescribed drugs or one specifically prescribed, usually by the anaesthetist.

Should patients take their normal drugs pre-operatively?

Yes. Most drugs can be taken with a sip of water. Exceptions include hypoglycaemic drugs and oral anticoagulants. Corticosteroid doses may need to be adjusted and/or intravenous administration considered.

Why might an anaesthetist prescribe pre-medication?

- To reduce anxiety and cause amnesia:
  - benzodiazepines (e.g. temazepam, midazolam) are most commonly used for this purpose. They also cause a degree of anterograde amnesia
- As pre-emptive analgesia:
  - analgesic pre-medication has been shown to reduce post-operative analgesic requirements. Commonly used drugs include paracetamol, NSAIDs and morphine
  - peripheral nerve blocks or regional anaesthesia can also be used
- As antiemetic:
  - pre-emptive antiemetics reduce post-operative nausea and vomiting. Cyclizine and metoclopramide are commonly used
- To increase gastric emptying and increase pH of gastric contents:

- pregnant women and patients with a history of hiatus hernia or with a full stomach are at a risk of vomiting or regurgitation during anaesthetic induction. Metoclopramide is used to enhance gastric emptying and ranitidine to raise gastric content pH
- To reduce secretions:
  - atropine or hyoscine is sometimes used to reduce secretions associated with certain types of anaesthetic agents, especially in children
- To reduce risk of peri-operative myocardial ischaemia in patients with ischaemic heart disease:
  - Beta adrenoreceptor blockers, e.g. atenolol can reduce the risk of intra- and post-operative cardiovascular complications

■ Pre-operative Investigations

What are the indications for performing blood investigations pre-operatively?

- Full blood count:
  - all women
  - all men over the age of 50
  - any haematological disorder
  - any significant past medical history
  - patients taking anticoagulant drugs
  - as a baseline measurement in surgery which will result in blood loss
- Urea and electrolytes:
  - age > 65
  - diabetes mellitus
  - any significant past medical history, e.g. renal or liver disease
  - patients with bowel obstruction
  - patients with vomiting or diarrhoea
  - any medication that can cause electrolyte imbalance, e.g. diuretics, digoxin, ACE inhibitors, corticosteroids, lithium
- Clotting screen:
  - liver disease
  - bleeding disorders
  - patients taking anticoagulant drugs
- Liver function tests:
  - liver disease
  - excess alcohol consumption (>50 units/ week)
- Glucose:
  - diabetes mellitus

- obesity
- patients taking corticosteroids
- Sickle cell screening:
  - patients who are from or whose parents are from African, Caribbean or Mediterranean countries
- Cross-matching:
  - most hospitals have a policy for each operation

Which patients should have a routine electrocardiogram (ECG) prior to surgery?

- Age >50
- Any patient with a cardiac history or on cardiac medications
- Any patient with a systemic disease associated with cardiac disorders, e.g. hypertension, diabetes mellitus, rheumatic fever, hyperlipidaemia
- Anyone undergoing a cardiothoracic operation

What are the indications for performing radiographs pre-operatively?

- Chest X-ray:
  - acute respiratory symptoms
  - known history of respiratory disease
  - any history of malignancy
  - perforated viscus
  - immigrants from TB endemic areas
  - cardiothoracic surgery
  - major upper abdominal surgery
  - thyroid enlargement
- Cervical spine X-ray: patients with rheumatoid arthritis who complain of neck pain or have reduced neck movements. These patients have an increased incidence of atlanto-axial subluxation, which can potentially cause spinal cord compression during intubation. Fibreoptic intubation is often required.

- Thoracic inlet X-ray: if tracheal compression or deviation is suspected, e.g. in patients with large goitres with retrosternal extension

Which patients should have a routine mid stream urine (MSU) sample taken prior to surgery?

Anyone undergoing joint replacement surgery or urological surgery.

Which patients will require tests of pulmonary function pre-operatively?

- Patients with chronic obstructive airway disease, lung fibrosis or severe asthma
- Patients with significant musculoskeletal abnormalities
- Patients undergoing thoracic surgery (to determine respiratory reserve prior to consideration for lung resection)

How may a patient with an established or suspected cardiac disease be investigated to determine the extent of the disease?

- Exercise ECG: economical method of assessing coronary artery disease; patients have to be able to exercise to a required rate
- Thallium scintigraphy: highly sensitive and specific in diagnosing coronary artery disease
- Echocardiogram: assesses left ventricular function
- Coronary angiogram: gold standard means of assessing cardiac function. It can be preceded with therapeutic interventional procedures such as angioplasty or stenting

■ Preparation for Surgery

What do asepsis and antisepsis mean?
Asepsis means no organisms are present during surgery. Antisepsis means total abolition of organisms has not been achieved and therefore some organisms will be present during surgery.

What is the difference between resident and transient bacterial flora?
Resident flora includes organisms that are present in the normal population, e.g. coagulase-negative staphylococci and corynebacteria.

Transient flora are organisms that are only consistently isolated from the skin of health care workers and are not always found in the normal population, e.g. *Staphylococcus aureus* and methicillin-resistant *Staphylococcus aureus* (MRSA).

What is the purpose of the surgical hand scrub?
- To remove dirt from the nails, hands and forearms
- To reduce resident and transient flora levels
- To prevent fast re-growth of bacteria

What property is essential in the antimicrobial agent used for the surgical hand scrub?
Organisms proliferate in the moist environment created by wearing of gloves and therefore antimicrobial agents must have persistent action to inhibit bacterial growth. Such agents include chlorhexidine gluconate and iodophors.

How should hair be removed pre-operatively?

- Depilatory cream should be used as it is associated with reduced wound infection rates
- If shaving or clipping is used, it should be done immediately before surgery to prevent bacterial colonisation of skin nicks

What precaution should be taken when using alcohol based agents in patient preparation?

The use of alcohol-based agents with diathermy can cause skin burns.

What properties should operating gowns possess?

They should:

- be comfortable
- provide a barrier to bacteria
- be impermeable to fluids
- minimise sweating
- be inexpensive

How may surgical drapes be a cause of wound infection?

The plastic adhesive strip attaching the drapes to the patient has been shown to increase wound infection rates. This is probably because sweating that occurs under the strips provides an environment for bacteria to grow.

Prostate Cancer

What are the risk factors for the development of prostate cancer?

- Age: increase in incidence over the age of 60
- Geographical distribution: highest incidence in North America and northern Europe; lowest incidence in the Far East
- Race: increased incidence in Afro-Americans and Afro-Caribbeans
- Family history: about 5–10% of cases are familial; if one first-degree relative affected risk increases by 2–3×
- Dietary: increased risk if diet high in fat, meat or Vitamin A
- High alcohol intake

Briefly describe the pathology of prostate cancer

- Adenocarcinoma (95%); transitional cell carcinoma (4%); rare types (neuro-endocrine carcinomas, sarcoma) (1%)
- Adenocarcinoma arises from glandular epithelium of the acinus in the posterior part of the gland; 70% from the peripheral zone, 20% from transitional and 10% from the central zone
- Prostatic intraepithelial neoplasia (PIN) may be a precursor to invasive prostatic cancer
- Local spread through capsule into perineural spaces, bladder neck, pelvic wall and rectum
- Lymphatic spread to obturator, iliac, pre-sacral and para-aortic nodes
- Haematogenous spread to lumbar spine, proximal femur, pelvis, ribs, skull and sternum; bony lesions are sclerotic on X-rays

- Histology described according to Gleason grading system. As most prostate cancers are heterogenous, the two predominant grades in a tumour are combined into a 'Gleason score' out of 10 to provide useful prognostic information

Gleason score	Description	Risk of progression over 10 years (%)
<4	Well differentiated	25
5–7	Moderately differentiated	50
>7	Poorly differentiated	75

How do prostate cancers clinically present?
- About 50% identified by PSA testing before patient becomes symptomatic
- Symptoms of bladder outflow obstruction including urinary retention
- Symptoms from metastases: bone pain, pathological fractures, cord compression, anaemia, weight loss
- Incidental finding in men undergoing TURP

Which investigations may be useful in the diagnosis of prostate cancers?
- Digital rectal examination: asymmetrical gland, loss of median sulcus, hard/craggy nodule, extension beyond the prostate, fixity
- Prostatic specific antigen (PSA): a glycoprotein responsible for liquefaction of semen, normal levels < 4 ng/ml; if levels are:

• 4–10 ng/ml	20–30% risk of cancer
• 10–20 ng/ml	50–75% risk
• >20 ng/ml	90% risk
• > 40 ng/ml	suggestive of lymph node or bone metastases

- Transrectal ultrasound (TRUS) and prostate biopsy
- Metastatic work-up:
  - bone scan and serum alkaline phosphatase: bony secondaries
  - MRI: extracapsular spread and seminal vesicle invasion
  - CT: lymph node involvement

Apart from prostate cancer what are the causes of an elevated PSA?

- Infection: UTI or prostatitis
- Benign prostatic hypertrophy (BPH)
- Urinary retention
- TURP
- Ejaculation
- Instrumentation: catheterisation, cystoscopy

What is the role of screening in prostate cancer?

- Although prostate cancer is a significant health problem and early detection could potentially lead to reduced morbidity and prolonged survival, it does not fulfil the other WHO criteria for population screening
- At the moment, there is no single, effective screening test for early prostate cancer in healthy men. PSA alone is used in the USA for men >50 or men >45 thought to be at high risk of prostate cancer. PSA alone is not recommended for screening in the UK because:
  - men with prostate cancer may not have a raised PSA (especially in early disease); conversely two out of three men with a raised PSA do not have prostate cancer
  - there is no consensus on the PSA level above which to commence treatment
  - two-thirds of men with a raised PSA level would go on to have unnecessary biopsies with its associated risks (pain,

per-rectal bleeding, haematuria, haemospermia, infection)
- there is uncertainty about the best way to treat early prostate cancer
- screening may detect slow growing tumours that may never present clinically

What are the treatment options in the management of prostate cancer?

Treatment is dependent on the stage of disease at presentation, grade of tumour, patient age and co-existing conditions.

For early staged, localised disease:
- watchful waiting: may be useful in elderly asymptomatic patients with a Gleason score < 5 or in patients not suitable for surgery. PSA monitored every 6 months and hormonal treatment considered if PSA shows a rising trend
- radiotherapy: usually indicated in patients with absence of lower urinary tract symptoms and who are unsuitable for surgery
- brachytherapy: implantation of radioactive seeds directly into the prostate under ultrasound control
- radical prostatectomy: *en bloc* resection of prostate, seminal vesicles ± obturator and pelvic nodes. Can be performed laparoscopically or through an open procedure (retropubic or perineal approach). Offers the best opportunity for a cure; however, there are significant risks associated with the procedure (impotence, incontinence, urethral stricture)

For locally advanced disease:
- watchful waiting: may be an option in elderly asymptomatic patients with a short life expectancy
- hormone treatment ± radiotherapy or radical prostatectomy

For metastatic disease:

- hormone treatment: based on medical or surgical androgen ablation; modes of treatment are blockade of androgen production in the:
  - hypothalamus–pituitary axis, e.g. goserelin, stilboestrol, cyproterone acetate
  - adrenal gland, e.g. ketoconazole, aminogluthetimide
  - prostate, e.g. flutamide, cyproterone acetate
  - testis: bilateral subcapsular orchidectomy
- for bone metastases: analgesics or localised radiotherapy to the affected region

■ Pyrexia

Define pyrexia

It is the elevation of body temperature above normal body temperature of 37.4 °C.

What are the common causes of post-operative pyrexia?

They can be summarised according to the post-operative time period in which they occur.

Post-operative period	Cause of pyrexia
0–24 h	systemic response to surgical trauma
24–72 h	atelectasis, pneumonia
3–7 days	pneumonia, wound infection, urinary tract infection, abdominal collection, anastomotic leak
7–10 days	DVT, PE, late wound infection

What is the management of the patient with post-operative pyrexia?

- Obtain detailed history:
  - cough
  - sputum
  - dysuria
  - calf pain
  - abdominal pain
- Thorough clinical examination:
  - cardiovascular: heart rate, blood pressure

- respiratory: elevated respiratory rate, breathlessness, crepitations
- abdominal: distension, signs of ileus
- wound: erythema, swelling, warmth, tenderness, discharge, dehiscence
- calves: swelling, erythema, warmth, tenderness
- Check vital signs:
  - temperature (check trend, e.g. persistently elevated, spikes)
  - cardiovascular: heart rate, blood pressure, urine output
  - respiratory: respiratory rate, oxygen saturation
  - central nervous system: GCS
- Investigations:
  - ECG
  - bloods: WCC, U and Es, CRP, ESR, blood cultures
  - mid stream urine: dipstick (should also be sent for microscopy and culture)
  - chest X-ray
  - arterial blood gases: metabolic acidosis, hypoxemia
  - doppler scan if DVT suspected
  - abdominal ultrasound or CT if abdominal collection suspected
  - spiral CT or ventilation–perfusion scan if PE suspected
- Treatment:

  All patients should receive adequate oxygenation and fluid resuscitation. Specific treatment is outlined below.

Condition	Treatment
Response to trauma	analgesics including paracetamol
Atelectasis	intensive chest physiotherapy, nebulised bronchodilators, antibiotics should only be given for associated infections
Pneumonia	chest physiotherapy, antibiotics as per hospital protocol

(cont.)

Condition	Treatment
Wound infection	antibiotics only once wound swab taken
Urinary tract infection	antibiotics only once MSU sample taken
Abdominal collection	broad spectrum antibiotics including anaerobic cover; collections should be drained
Anastomotic leak	radiologically or surgically; anastomotic leaks may require further surgery
DVT/PE	anticoagulants should be commenced as soon as possible and must not be delayed until appropriate investigations are performed

■ Radiology

How can radiological techniques be used in the management of surgical diseases?

- They can aid in the diagnosis of surgical disorders:
  - acutely, e.g. diagnosis of fractures; CXR to detect intra-peritoneal gas
  - population screening, e.g. mammography
- As interventional techniques to treat a surgical problem
  - to obtain tissue samples, e.g. core breast biopsy using digital mammography
  - placement of drains, e.g. for abscesses under USS or CT guidance
  - interventional stenting of aneurysms
  - feeding, e.g. percutaneous gastrostomy
  - central venous access, e.g. for chemotherapy, TPN
  - embolisation, e.g. for skeletal metastases
  - vertebroplasty, e.g. for vertebral metastases
  - tumour ablation, e.g. hepatic, bone, soft tissue
- Image guided surgery:
  - X-ray, e.g. for treatment of fractures, ERCP
  - USS, e.g. during hepatic resections
  - CT, e.g. stereotactic neurosurgery
  - MRI, e.g. in neurosurgery

What are the advantages of interventional techniques compared with conventional surgery?

- Avoids general anaesthesia in most cases
- Most procedures can be performed as day cases resulting in shorter hospital stay
- Procedures are often more cost-effective
- Reduced morbidity post-procedure

■ Regional Anaesthesia

What are the two commonly used methods of achieving regional anaesthesia?

- Spinal anaesthesia: local anaesthetic or opiate administered into CSF below the cauda equina
- Epidural anaesthesia: local anaesthetic or opiate administered into the epidural space

What are the main differences between them?

	Spinals	Epidurals
• Onset of block:	rapid (<5 min)	slow (up to 30 min)
• Duration of action:	1–2 h	2–3 h
• Continuous infusion with catheter:	No	Yes
• Dose of local anaesthetic:	Small	Large

What are the main contraindications to their use?

- Coagulation disorders
- Neurological disorders
- Hypovolaemia
- Septicaemia

List some of their complications

- Immediate
  - hypotension (spinal > epidural)
  - high blockade

- Early
  - urinary retention (spinal > epidural)
  - backache
  - headache (spinal > epidural)
  - infection

Why does hypotension occur in regional anaesthesia?

The control of blood pressure is under the sympathetic nervous system. Sympathetic outflow from spinal cord occurs between T1 and L2. This is blocked to varying degrees in both spinal and epidural anaesthesia causing vasodilation and therefore hypotension. It is usually treated with fluid resuscitation and occasionally with sympathomimetic drugs such as ephedrine.

What is the incidence of dural tear in regional anaesthesia? What are the symptoms and how is it treated?

Incidence is up to 5% in spinal anaesthesia but much less common in epidurals. Symptoms include occipital headache which is exacerbated on standing up, nausea and vomiting. In most patients it resolves within a few days with bed rest, analgesia and fluids.

How should a patient be prepared before receiving a regional block?

Similar preparation is required as that for a general anaesthetic, i.e. pre-operative assessment with any relevant investigations performed.

Renal Failure and Surgery

What are the main causes of chronic renal failure?
- Diabetes mellitus
- Glomerulonephritis
- Chronic pyelonephritis
- Renal vascular disease
- Polycystic kidneys
- Drug induced

What are the systemic complications of chronic renal failure (CRF)?
- Cardiovascular:
  - hypertension
  - chronic anaemia (due to uraemia and ↓ erythropoietin levels)
  - peripheral vascular disease
- Acid–base disturbances:
  - metabolic acidosis
  - hyperkalaemia
  - hyponatraemia
  - hypocalcaemia
  - hypermagnesaemia
  - impaired water haemostasis
- Immunity
  - reduced phagocyte function
  - reduced immunity secondary to use of immunosuppressants
- Gastrointestinal:
  - reflux oesophagitis
  - gastric erosions and peptic ulceration

- Coagulation:
  - coagulopathy: ↓ platelet adhesiveness which increases bleeding time
- Endocrine:
  - diabetes mellitus
  - hyperparathyroidism
- Musculoskeletal
  - osteoporosis
  - osteomalacia
  - pathological fractures

What are the particular risks of anaesthesia in patients with CRF?

- Presence of vascular access fistulae for haemodialysis may limit sites for venous access
- Intra-operative hypotension can cause clotting of fistulae
- Anaesthesia within 6 hours of haemodialysis can cause cardiovascular instability (due to fluid shifts between compartments)
- Administration of anaesthetic agents, e.g. suxamethonium can worsen the hyperkalaemia
- Increased bleeding time presents an increased risk of spinal haematoma therefore regional anaesthesia may be unsuitable

What are the indications for urgent dialysis pre-operatively?

- Fluid overload
- Hyperkalaemia
- Severe metabolic acidosis
- Severe uraemia

Respiratory Disease and Surgery

Why are patients with respiratory disease at increased risk of post-operative pulmonary complications?

They have impaired respiratory function due to:

- decreased lung compliance
- increased bronchial secretions
- bronchospasm
- superimposed infections

What symptoms should specifically be asked about when taking a history from these patients?

- Dyspnoea
- Cough
- Sputum
  - colour
  - volume
- Need for home oxygen
- Smoking history
- Exercise tolerance
- Previous admission to ITU for ventilation

What may routine pre-operative investigations reveal in these patients?

- Blood tests:
  - elevated haemoglobin levels secondary to polycythaemia
  - elevated white cell count secondary to acute infections
- ECG:
  - right heart strain
  - ischaemic changes

- Chest X-ray:
  - tracheal deviation
  - lung disease
  - cardiomegaly

What specific tests may be useful in optimising pre-operative care?
- Arterial blood gases:
  - elevated $PaCO_2$ concentrations indicate increased probability of post-operative pulmonary complications including need for post-operative ventilation
- Sputum culture and sensitivity will allow successful treatment of any infective exacerbations
- Lung function tests:
  - patients with reduced FEV_1 : FVC ratios have significantly higher incidence of postoperative complications which can be reduced considerably with appropriate pre-operative management

What measures can be taken to optimise these patients in the pre-operative period?
- Smoking should be stopped at least 4 months before surgery but even cessation 48 h prior to surgery is associated with reduced complication rates
- Aggressive physiotherapy to clear secretions and thus improve lung function
- Antibiotics to treat acute exacerbations
- Nebulised bronchodilators to reduce bronchospasm
- Corticosteroids to reduce associated inflammation

What anaesthetic considerations need to be taken into account?
- Regional anaesthesia should be considered whenever possible

- General anaesthesia may need to be supplemented with intermittent positive pressure ventilation
- In patients with bullous disease, positive pressure ventilation or the use of nitrous oxide can rupture bullae, leading to tension pneumothorax

What considerations need to be taken into account in the post-operative period?

- Patients may require ventilatory support and this should have been identified and planned for in the pre-operative period
- Humidified oxygen should be administered to prevent viscous secretions
- Patients should be nursed in an upright position to optimise residual capacity
- Adequate analgesia administered to allow deep breathing and early mobilisation
- Chest physiotherapy to clear secretions and reduce basal airway closure
- Advice and support given regarding cessation of smoking

Rheumatoid Arthritis

What are the non-operative methods for treating rheumatoid arthritis?

- Patient education: regarding the need for lifestyle changes to prevent exacerbations, to preserve mobility and functionality, and for appropriate pain management
- Drugs
  - first-line treatment, e.g. NSAIDs
  - second-line treatment, e.g. corticosteroids, chloroquine, penicillamine
  - third-line treatment, e.g. immunosuppressants
- Rest and immobilisation: this will reduce joint swelling and can induce disease remission. Rest may require hospital admission
- Physiotherapy: to restore joint movements especially after an acute attack
- Walking aids
- Splints and braces to protect painful joints
- Specialised footwear to relieve strain on pressure areas
- Intra-articular steroid injections

What are the indications for surgery in patients with rheumatoid arthritis?

For articular disease:

- synovectomy: can minimise flare-ups and slow down disease progression when medical treatment has failed
- arthroplasty: for advanced disease of the larger joints
- arthrodesis: for disease affecting the smaller joints

For extra-articular manifestations:
- atlanto-axial instability
- extensor tendon ruptures at the wrist
- popliteal cysts
- carpal tunnel syndrome
- splenomegaly (in patients with Felty syndrome)

■ Scars

What is the difference between hypertrophic and keloid scars?

In hypertrophic scars, the excess scar tissue is limited to the site of the original wound. They occur due to over-activity in the proliferative phase of wound healing. They usually self-correct within a year and a normal scar forms.

In keloid scars, the excess scar tissue extends beyond the original wound. They occur due to intense fibroblast over-activity into the remodelling phase of wound healing. They do not self correct.

What are the predisposing factors for keloid scar formation?

- Young age
- Males
- Afro-Caribbean race

What are the most common sites for keloid scar formation?

- Sternum
- Shoulders and upper arms
- Head and neck

How can keloid scar formation be minimised?

- Incisions should run parallel to skin tension lines
- Tension free wound closure
- Prevention of wound infection and haematomas

What are the treatment options for keloid scars?
- Compression garments
- Silastic gel therapy
- Steroid injection into the scar
- Scar excision
- Radiotherapy
- Laser therapy

Why do contractures occur?
They occur when a scar shortens resulting in reduced tissue and/or joint mobility. It is mainly due to poor surgical technique in wound closure. They often require further surgery including skin grafting.

■ Screening

What are the principles of a national screening programme?

The condition:

- should be an important health problem
- and its natural history from preclinical stage to established condition should be detectable and prevalent
- should have a latent stage (if early detection does not improve outcome there is no benefit from screening)

The test should be:

- such that it has a high:
  - sensitivity (proportion of those with disease who test positive)
  - specificity (proportion of those without disease who test negative)
  - Positive Predictive Value (PPV): the likelihood that a positive test result indicates the existence of the disease
  - Negative Predictive Value (NPV): the likelihood that a negative test result indicates the absence of the disease
  - reliability: the ability of a test to give consistent results when performed more than once on the same individual under the same conditions
- acceptable to the population
- inexpensive
- accurate

The treatment:

- should be effective with evidence of early treatment leading to better outcomes than late treatment
- should be agreed, i.e. there should be a policy on who to treat for the condition and patient outcomes should be optimised

in all health care providers prior to participation in a
screening programme

The screening programme:

- should be derived from high quality Randomised Controlled
  Trials and be effective in reducing mortality or morbidity
- when aimed at providing information to allow the person
  being screened to make an 'informed choice' (e.g. Down's
  syndrome), there must be evidence that the test accurately
  measures risk
- and its implications must be understood by the individual
  being screened.
- should be clinically, socially and ethically acceptable to
  health professionals and the public
- benefits should outweigh the physical and psychological
  harm (caused by the test, diagnostic procedures and
  treatment)

What are the adverse effects of screening?

- Consequences of a false positive result:
  - anxiety and stress
  - unnecessary investigation and treatment
- Consequences of a false-negative result:
  - can have tragic implications
  - false sense of security which may delay final diagnosis
  - patients might neglect future screening tests

What are the different biases associated with screening?

Bias is any systematic error that affects the evaluation of a
screening test performance. These can be:

- lead time bias: the apparently better survival observed for
  those screened is not because these patients are actually
  living longer, but instead because diagnosis is being made at
  an earlier point in the natural history of the disease

- over-diagnosis bias:
  - enthusiasm for a new screening program may result in higher rates of false-positives and give false impression of increased rates of diagnosis and detection
  - screening may identify abnormalities that would never cause a problem in a person's lifetime, e.g. autopsy studies have shown that a high proportion of men who have died in other ways, have prostate cancer
  - benign or indolent conditions are often detected
- selection bias: not everyone will partake in a screening programme; there are factors that differ between those willing to get tested and those who are not, e.g.
  - if people with a higher risk of a disease are more eager to be screened (e.g. women with a family history of breast cancer joining a mammography programme), then a screening test will look worse than it really is because there are going to be more people with the illness joining, and a higher chance of people dying of that illness
  - if a test is more available to young and healthy people (for instance, if people have to travel a long distance to get checked), then fewer people in the screening population will become ill, and the test will seem to make a positive difference, thus making the test look better than it really is
- length bias: screening detects less aggressive cancers with long preclinical phases (and better prognoses)

What are the barriers to screening?
Patient barriers:
- social and cultural norms
- psychological factors (fear and anxiety)
- behavioural factors
- perceptions of personal risk for disease

Physician barriers
- lack of time
- mobile populations: documentation and follow-up difficult
- lack of professional consensus on benefits of some screening tests

List three cancers for which there are established national screening programmes
- Breast: mammography
- Cervical: Pap test
- Colorectal: faecal occult blood

■ Sedation

What is the aim of sedation?
It is to achieve a reduced level of consciousness whilst retaining verbal communication with the patient. It is used to reduce pain and anguish during certain diagnostic and interventional procedures.

List the advantages and disadvantages of sedation
Advantages:
- avoids general anaesthesia
- allows certain procedures to be performed in patients who are unsuitable for general anaesthesia
- retains communication with the patient, which may be important in certain procedures
- provides amnesia
- quicker recovery from the procedure

Disadvantages:
- drug overdose can cause respiratory depression and loss of consciousness
- does not provide pain relief and often opiates have to be added. The combined effect of these two agents can cause respiratory depression

Which drugs are commonly used to achieve sedation?
Benzodiazepines, e.g. midazolam or diazepam

Can the effects of these drugs be reversed?
Yes. Flumazenil is a specific benzodiazepine antagonist. Limitations to its use include a short duration of action with the potential for re-sedation; it can cause convulsions and is expensive

What precautions are mandatory before administering sedation?

- Intravenous access
- Oxygen
- Full resuscitation facilities including resuscitation drugs
- Use only a table or trolley that can be tipped down
- Ensure adequate help is available if needed

Do patients undergoing sedation need to be monitored?

Yes. Patients must be monitored (pulse oximetry, blood pressure and ECG) throughout and after the procedure until they are fully conscious and their vital signs are stable.

Which group of patients are at particular risk during sedation?

- Children
- Elderly
- Obese
- Patients with co-existing cardiorespiratory disease
- Patients with gastrointestinal bleeding

■ Sickle Cell Disease

What is sickle cell disease?

An abnormality of haemoglobin synthesis, which results in increased rigidity of red cells (sickling) with a reduced survival (haemolytic anaemia) and obstruction of the microcirculation. Sickling (crisis) is often precipitated by infection, dehydration, cold or hypoxia. When only the trait is present, the red cells do not usually sickle until the oxygen saturation falls below 40%, which is rarely reached in venous blood.

Why should surgeons know something about sickle cell disease?

- Common surgical conditions occur in sickle cell patients and surgery in these patients can be associated with increased morbidity and mortality
- Some surgical conditions are more common in sickle cell patients:
  - abdominal pain during a crisis
  - hepatosplenomegaly
  - hepatic and splenic infarction
  - pigment gallstones
  - bone pain and bone infarction during a crisis
  - avascular necrosis of bone
  - dactylitis
  - joint effusions
  - salmonella osteomyelitis
  - haematuria
  - priapism

What are the principles of surgery in these patients?

Pre-operatively:

- patients who are from, or whose parents are from, African, Caribbean or Mediterranean countries should be screened for sickle cell status if it is not known
- assessment should centre on signs and symptoms of end-organ damage, e.g. cor pulmonale, liver disease and renal failure
- prolonged fasting and dehydration should be avoided as they can precipitate a crisis
- blood transfusion may be required to reduce HbS to less than 30% of total Hb without increasing the haematocrit above 36%

Operatively:

- avoid factors which precipitate a crisis:
  - preoxygenation with optimised oxygenation
  - adequate fluid replacement with avoidance of hypotension
  - warming devices and increase in operating theatre temperature to avoid hypothermia
- tourniquets should be avoided but if their use is essential then minimise the inflation period

Post-operatively:

- oxygen therapy should be continued for at least 24 h post-surgery
- regular chest physiotherapy as pulmonary complications are common
- strong analgesia is essential
- regular examination of patients as crises can occur during surgery and symptoms can be concealed by anaesthesia and analgesia
- high dependency care may be required after major surgery
- be aware that a crisis can manifest as the acute chest syndrome (chest wall pain, fever, cough, hypoxia and pulmonary infiltrates) which has a high mortality rate

▪ Small Bowel Obstruction

What are the causes of small bowel obstruction?

- Causes within the lumen:
  - faecal impaction
  - gallstone 'ileus'
  - foreign body
  - meconium ileus
- Causes in the lumen wall:
  - Crohn's disease
  - primary bowel tumour
  - diverticulitis
  - congenital atresia
- Causes outside the lumen wall:
  - adhesions
  - strangulated hernia
  - volvulus
  - intussusception

Of these, which are most common causes of small bowel obstruction in the UK?

- Adhesions
- Strangulated hernia
- Malignancy

Briefly describe the pathophysiology of intestinal obstruction

The bowel proximal to the obstructing lesion becomes dilated with swallowed air and intestinal fluid. In an attempt to overcome the obstruction there is increased peristalsis resulting in intestinal colic. Dilation of the gut wall produces mucosal oedema which impairs blood flow resulting in intestinal ischaemia. In severe cases, infarction and perforation ensues. The overall effects are dehydration with electrolyte imbalance (due to vomiting and loss into the bowel lumen) and systemic toxicity (due to toxins and intestinal bacteria escaping into the peritoneal cavity through ischaemic or perforated bowel).

What are the clinical features of small bowel obstruction?

Symptoms:
- colicky abdominal pain: usually in the peri-umbilical region and occurs with greater frequency in high small bowel than in low small bowel obstruction
- vomiting: occurs early in high small obstruction and late in small bowel obstruction. In late stages of small bowel obstruction the vomiting becomes faeculent due to accumulation of bacteria which begin to decompose the stagnant contents of the obstructed small bowel
- abdominal distention: this is marked in low small bowel obstruction and may be minimal in high small bowel obstruction
- absolute constipation: a late feature of small bowel obstruction

Signs:
- on inspection:
  - dehydration with associated tachycardia, hypotension and oliguria
  - visible peristalsis may be present in some cases
  - assessed for a strangulated hernia
- on palpation: generalised abdominal tenderness
- on auscultation: high pitched bowel sounds with associated borborygmi

Which investigations may be useful in the management of small bowel obstruction?

- Bloods: WCC, U and Es
- Arterial blood gases: metabolic acidosis
- Abdominal X-ray:
  - small bowel differentiated from large bowel by valvulae coniventes
  - distended small bowel loops present centrally
  - absent or minimal colonic gas
- Small bowel contrast study: this can be either a follow through study or a small bowel enema
- CT: useful in determining the cause of obstruction and distinguishes between ileus and mechanical small bowel obstruction in post-operative patients

Describe the initial management of small bowel obstruction

- Patients should be kept nil by mouth with administration of intravenous analgesia and anti-emetic agents
- Aggressive fluid resuscitation with intravenous saline and potassium. Adequacy of resuscitation can be determined by urine output and/or central venous pressure monitoring
- Placement of a naso-gastric tube which:
  - decompresses the bowel
  - stops vomiting
  - prevents the risk of aspiration during induction of anaesthesia
  - aids in monitoring fluid losses from the G.I. tract
- Antibiotics to cover gram negative and anaerobic organisms if perforation is suspected
- Appropriate investigations (outlined above) performed

What are the indications for non-surgical treatment of small bowel obstruction?

Conservative treatment with iv fluids and naso-gastric aspiration ('drip and suck') is only indicated when:

- obstruction is thought to be due to adhesions and there are no features of peritonism. Patients should be reviewed regularly and if there is any deterioration in the clinical condition, an urgent laparotomy should be considered
- the distinction from post-surgical paralytic ileus is uncertain and a period of observation is indicated

What are the indications for surgery in a patient with small bowel obstruction?

- Obstruction in the absence of previous abdominal surgery ('virgin' abdomen)
- Strangulated hernia
- Peritonitis
- Failed trial of conservative treatment

How can the viability of bowel be determined intra-operatively?

Non-viability can be assessed by the loss of:

- peristalsis
- colour (green or black bowel)
- mesenteric arterial pulsation

Bowel of doubtful viability should be wrapped in warm wet packs and reassessed after a few minutes. If deemed viable, it can be returned to the abdominal cavity; otherwise it should be resected.

What do you understand by the term paralytic ileus?

Paralytic ileus is a functional obstruction of the small bowel due to reduced intestinal motility. Aetiology includes recent abdominal surgery, trauma, intestinal ischaemia, sepsis, hypokalaemia, and certain drugs, e.g. anticholinergic agents. The main clinical features are abdominal distention, absolute constipation and vomiting. In contrast with mechanical obstruction, pain is not a prominent feature (due to the absence of peristalsis); bowel sounds are absent, whereas accentuated bowel sounds indicate mechanical obstruction; symptoms usually subside within 4–5 days; and abdominal X-rays may show a diffuse gas pattern as opposed to a localised distended bowel loop seen in mechanical obstruction. If diagnosis remains uncertain, small bowel contrast studies or a CT scan can help in distinguishing between the two conditions. Management includes minimal handling of bowel at time of surgery, correction of any electrolyte disturbances, treatment of underlying sepsis, administration of IV fluids and placement of a naso-gastric tube. At present, there is no proven medical treatment available. The condition usually resolves spontaneously within a few days.

■ Smoking

What are the adverse physiological effects of tobacco smoke?

- Cardiovascular:
  - nicotine increases myocardial workload and oxygen requirements
  - nicotine acts as a potent adrenergic agonist producing an increase in blood pressure, heart rate and systemic vascular resistance
  - nicotine and carbon monoxide alter myocardial electrophysiology, lowering the threshold for arrhythmias
  - carbon monoxide combines with haemoglobin to form carboxyhaemoglobin (COHb) which decreases the available oxygen that is transported to tissues
  - carbon monoxide has a negative inotropic effect
- Respiratory:
  - hyper-secretion of mucus and ciliary dysfunction resulting in impaired tracheobronchial clearance and sputum retention
  - small airway narrowing

What are the potential problems of surgery in patients who smoke?

Pre-operatively:
- patients are more likely to have associated medical problems:
  - cardiovascular: hypertension, coronary artery disease, peripheral vascular disease, hyperlipidaemia
  - respiratory: chronic obstructive pulmonary disease
  - gastrointestinal: peptic ulcer disease

- endocrine: diabetes mellitus
- haematological: polycythaemia, increased platelet aggregability
- immune: impaired immunity
- smoking can affect the metabolism of certain drugs, e.g. theophylline, warfarin, propanolol
- general anaesthesia requirements (especially thiopentone) are higher in smokers
- high COHb levels interfere with the accuracy of pulse oximeters, e.g. in a patient with 10% COHb, the pulse oximeter may display a saturation of 100%, when in fact the actual saturation is 90%

Operatively:
- less successful outcomes following certain types of surgery, e.g. following spinal fusion, arterial reconstructions and skin grafting

Post-operatively: smokers have a higher incidence of:
- respiratory complications: basal lung collapse, atelectasis, hypoxia, pneumonia
- wound infections and wound dehiscence
- incisional hernias
- increased analgesic requirements
- deep venous thrombosis
- readmissions to hospital, mainly due to pulmonary complications

Are there any benefits of pre-operative smoking cessation in the short term?

Yes. Even patients who stop smoking within 12 to 24 hours before surgery will at least improve some cardiac functioning due to carbon monoxide and nicotine elimination. Smoking cessation in the short-term results in improvement in ciliary function (2–7 days); reduction in sputum volume (1–2 weeks); improvement of small airway narrowing with significant uction in post-operative complications (4–6 weeks); and improved immune function (6–8 weeks).

Splenectomy

http://www.surgical-tutor.org.uk/default-home.htm?core/trauma/spleen. htmñight

http://www.emedicine.com/med/topic2792.htm

http://www.nordictraumarad.com/splenic%20injury%20Huddinge% 20Trauma%20manual%200411.pdf

http://www.emedicine.com/RADIO/topic645.htm

Staging of Tumours

What do you understand by the terms grading and staging of tumours?

Grading is the assessment of the degree of differentiation and the number of mitosis within the tumour. In general, higher-grade tumours are more aggressive than lower-grade tumours. Grading has restrictive value because different parts of the same tumour may display different degrees of differentiation and the grade of tumour may change as the tumour grows.

Staging is based on the anatomic extent of the tumour. Relevant to staging are the size of the primary tumour and the extent of local and distant spread. It is based on clinical, radiological, histological and surgical information. Staging has been proved to be of greater prognostic value than tumour grading.

What properties should a 'perfect' staging system possess?

It should be:
- simple to remember and use
- reproducible: not subject to inter- or intra-observer variation
- based on a small number of prognostically important parameters

What are the advantages of having a staging system?

- It provides useful information regarding prognosis
- It allows decisions to be made regarding adjuvant therapy
- Comparisons can be made regarding treatment outcomes between different centres

List three staging systems that are commonly used in clinical practice

TNM system: T refers to the extent of the primary tumour; N refers to the extent of regional lymph node spread; and M refers to the presence or absence of distant metastasis. The addition of numbers to the letters indicates the extent of spread in each category. For example, in breast carcinoma:

- T – primary tumour
  - T_0: cannot be assessed clinically
  - T_1: <2 cm
  - T_2: >2 cm but <5 cm
  - T_3: >5 cm
  - T_4: any size with chest wall or skin extension
- N – regional lymph nodes
  - N_0: no node metastasis
  - N_1: ipsilateral axillary (mobile)
  - N_2: ipsilateral axillary (fixed)
  - N_3: ipsilateral internal mammary nodes
- M – distant metastasis
  - M_0: no distant metastasis
  - M_1: distant metastasis present

Dukes' ABC system: devised for rectal carcinomas but is now used for rectal and colonic carcinomas. The classification has been modified to include two 'B' and 'C' categories as well as a 'D' category to represent distant metastases.

Stage	Definition	5-year survival (%)
A	Spread to submucosa but not muscle	90
B	Spread to muscle but node negative	70
C	Lymph node metastases present	40

In malignant melanoma, the most important prognostic factor is tumour thickness. The most commonly used staging system involves the depth of invasion by Breslow thickness measured from the granular layer of the epidermis to the deepest point of tumour infiltration in the vertical dimension. In the absence of satellite or lymph-node involvement, the 5-year survival is:

Depth (mm)	5-year survival (%)
<0.75	9–99
0.76–1.49	8–90
1.50–3.99	6–75
>4.0	<50

■ Stomas

What is a stoma?
When any part of the gastrointestinal tract is brought to the surface and opened it is called a stoma.

How can stomas be classified?
- Temporary or permanent:
  - temporary stomas, e.g. oesophagostomy, loop ileostomy, caecostomy
  - permanent stomas, e.g. end colostomy, end ileostomy
- By use:
  - enteral feeding, e.g. gastrostomy, jejunostomy
  - decompression, e.g. caecostomy to decompress the large bowel
  - diversion, e.g. faecal stream diversion as in a loop ileostomy after AP resection or oesophagostomy to divert food material from the bronchial tree
  - lavage of bowel contents

Where should a stoma be located?
The position of a stoma should be discussed between the patient and a specialist stoma nurse and its location marked pre-operatively. The location should be in the most favourable position for the patient, away from any bony prominences and in a position which is easy for the patient to manage.

What are the complications of a stoma?
- Immediate:
  - bleeding
  - ischaemia (usually due to technical failure)

- Early:
  - high output
  - obstruction
  - retraction
- Late:
  - obstruction
  - prolapse
  - herniation
  - skin excoriation
  - skin hypersensitivity
  - psychiatric morbidity

How can a colostomy be differentiated from an ileostomy?

An end colostomy is usually located in the left iliac fossa, whereas a transverse colostomy is normally located in the right or left upper quadrants. An ileostomy is usually located in the right iliac fossa. In a colostomy, the bowel mucosa is usually flush with the skin whereas an ileostomy has a spout (to prevent skin excoriation from the discharging fluid).

■ Sutures and Ligatures

What is the purpose of a suture?
It is to hold the wound in apposition until healing by primary intension occurs.

How would you choose a suture?
The smallest diameter suture that will adequately appose the wound should be used to limit tissue trauma and to reduce the quantity of foreign material retained within tissues.

Define suture 'memory'
Memory is the ability of a suture to return to its original shape or assume a new shape with use. It is directly related to the elastic properties of the suture. Sutures with good memory, e.g. Nylon and PDS are more difficult to handle and have poor knot qualities compared with sutures with no memory, e.g. silk.

List some general principles of tying a good knot
- Type of knot to be used should be appropriate to the suture material used
- Do not use excessive tension as this can fracture the suture
- Approximate – don't strangulate the tissues
- Too many throws will increases foreign body mass and predispose to stitch abscesses. In general use three throws for multifilament suture, four throws for monofilament suture and up to seven throws when using prolene
- Avoid holding the needle butt as it can cause needle and sutures to fracture

How are sutures classified?

- Absorbable or non-absorbable:
  - absorbable sutures can be monofilament or multifilament, natural or synthetic. They are broken down by either proteolysis (e.g. catgut) or hydrolysis (most synthetic sutures). They lose most of their strength within 60 days of application
- Monofilament or multifilament (braided):
  - monofilament sutures are smooth and easily incorporated into tissues but have poor knot qualities. Holding monofilament sutures with instruments can significantly reduce its tensile strength and even fracture the suture
  - multifilament sutures are easier to handle than monofilament sutures and have good knot characteristics. Disadvantage of use includes the fact that interstices of the suture can potentially become colonised with bacteria
- Natural or synthetic:
  - natural sutures induce a marked tissue inflammatory response

List some commonly used sutures with their properties

Suture	Material	Synthetic or natural	Monofilament or braided	Properties
Absorbable				
Catgut	Animal intestine	Natural	Monofilament	Absorbed by 90 days; strength retained for 3 weeks
Maxon	Polyglyconate	Synthetic	Monofilament	Absorbed by 200 days
PDS	Polydioxanone	Synthetic	Monofilament	Absorbed by 200 days; strength retained for 4 weeks
Dexon	Polyglycolic acid	Synthetic	Braided	Absorbed by 90 days (*cont.*)

(*Cont.*)

Suture	Material	Synthetic or natural	Monofilament or braided	Properties
Vicryl	Polylactin 910	Synthetic	Braided	Absorbed by 70 days; Tensile strength: 65% at 14 days 40% at 21 days 10% at 35 days
Non-absorbable				
Silk	Silkworm cocoons	Natural	Braided	Strength retained for several weeks
Prolene	Polypropylene	Synthetic	Monofilament	High tensile strength
Ethilon	Nylon-polyamide	Synthetic	Monofilament and braided	Good elasticity; has high memory
Ti-cron	Polyester	Synthetic	Monofilament and braided	Good handling characteristics; can cause tissue drag
Steel wire				Used to close sternotomy wounds

List some other methods of closing wounds

- Steristrips: suitable for superficial lacerations only and cannot be used if there is wound tension
- Tissue 'glue': polymerises rapidly when applied on the wound, forming a firm adhesive bond
- Stapling devices: commonly used in bowel anastomosis
- Skin clips: quick to use, produce a good scar and have lower incidence of infection but can be uncomfortable to the patient

Thyroid Surgery

Which investigations may be useful in the management of thyroid disease?

Blood tests:

- hormone measurements:
  - TSH: raised in hypothyroidism and reduced in hyperthyroidism
  - Free T4 and T3: raised levels in thyrotoxicosis
  - calcitonin: used in follow-up of patients who have undergone a thyroidectomy for medullary thyroid tumours
- autoantibodies:
  - anti-TPO: raised in Hahimoto's thyroiditis
  - thyroid stimulating immunoglobulin: raised in Grave's disease
- tumour markers:
  - thyroglobulin (Tg): following total thyroidectomy ± radioiodine ablation therapy for cancer, serum Tg levels should be <3–5 ng/ml; levels > 5 ng/ml are suggestive of residual disease and rising levels suggest recurrent disease

Imaging:

- ultrasound: does not reliably distinguish between benign and malignant lesions but may be used to:
  - distinguish between cystic and solid lesions
  - identify multinodularity
  - monitor progress of benign nodules
  - assess for lymphadenopathy
- CT: mainly used to assess retrosternal goitres, goitres with pressure symptoms or as part of pre-operative work-up in patients with cancer

- MRI: may be used to assess the degree of spread into the neck, mediastinum and cervical lymph nodes in patients with medullary or papillary cancers
- radionuclide scanning: provides information about thyroid function; scanning may reveal if a nodule is 'hot' (functional) or 'cold' (non-functional)

How can thyroid tumours be classified?
Benign:
- follicular adenoma
- papillary adenoma (rare)

Malignant:
- papillary carcinoma (most common)
- follicular carcinoma
- medullary carcinoma
- anaplastic (undifferentiated) carcinoma
- lymphoma
- Hürthle cell carcinoma
- metastases

Why is FNAC not useful in diagnosing a follicular carcinoma?
Unlike papillary carcinoma, cytology does not distinguish between follicular carcinoma and a follicular adenoma and therefore diagnosis is made histologically after resection.

What is the role of surgery in thyroid disease?
- Isthmusectomy:
  - solitary nodule confined to the isthmus
  - in anaplastic carcinoma or lymphoma to relieve tracheal compression
- Lobectomy and isthmusectomy:
  - solitary nodules
  - multinodular disease confined to one lobe

- Subtotal thyroidectomy:
  - Grave's disease following failed medical treatment in the young patient or in women who may become pregnant within 2 years of radioiodine treatment
  - multinodular goitre in both lobes
- Total thyroidectomy:
  - well differentiated and medullary carcinomas
  - Grave's disease: following failed medical treatment in the young patient; in women who may become pregnant within 2 years of radioiodine treatment; in patients with significant ophthalmopathy or very large goitres
  - multinodular goitres

What are the principles of thyroid surgery?

Pre-operatively:
- FNAC to confirm diagnosis
- CXR in all patients with suspected or proven cancers and in the presence of pressure symptoms
- CT or MRI in patients with extensive or recurrent disease
- patients should be rendered euthyroid and thyroid function tests and serum calcium recorded prior to surgery
- laryngoscopy to assess vocal cords: particularly important if recurrent laryngeal nerve palsy suspected or in revision surgery
- patient is positioned with the neck extended to allow adequate access. The table can be tilted head-up to increase venous return and reduce venous engorgement in the neck

Operatively:
- standard approach is via an open operation through a collar incision
- identify and protect the recurrent laryngeal nerve throughout the procedure
- parathyroid glands should be identified and preserved with their blood supply

- haemostasis is essential
- use of suction drain (optional)
- meticulous wound closure

Post-operatively:

- assess for bleeding: this is usually deep to the strap muscles and can lead to laryngeal oedema and airway obstruction. If bleeding suspected, the patient should be immediately returned to theatre for evacuation of haematoma and control of bleeding

What are the other complications of thyroid surgery?

- Nerve damage:
  - branches of the anterior cutaneous nerve of the face
  - external branch of superior laryngeal nerve (most commonly injured): damage can result in voice change especially noticed during singing
  - recurrent laryngeal nerve: if one nerve is damaged there may be voice hoarseness and reduced force whilst coughing; bilateral damage may cause stridor and airway obstruction
  - cervical sympathetic plexus: injury causes Horner's syndrome
- Hypocalcaemia: usually transient but may take up to 6 months to recover
- Hypothyroidism
- Thyroid crisis: usually as a result of inadequate pre-operative work-up
- Recurrent thyrotoxicosis: seen particularly after thyroidectomy for Grave's disease
- Tracheomalacia (rare)
- Keloid scarring

▪ Tourniquets

What are the benefits of tourniquet use?
- Reduction of blood loss therefore providing better operative visual field
- Prevention of drugs given in high doses into an isolated limb entering the systemic circulation during:
  - intravenous regional anaesthesia
  - isolated limb perfusion treatment for melanomas or soft tissue sarcomas in the extremities

What are the contraindications to the use of tourniquets?
- Peripheral vascular disease
- Previous vascular surgery on the limb the tourniquet is to be used on
- Past history of thrombo-embolic events
- Sickle cell disease (relative contraindication)
- Vasculitic disorders

What pressures should tourniquets be inflated to?
They are usually inflated to 100–150 mmHg above systolic blood pressure. In children, lower pressures should be used.

What is the maximum duration that tourniquets should be used for?
They should not be used for longer than 60 minutes for the upper limb and 90 minutes for the lower limb. Periodic deflation (about 10 min), followed by re-inflation can permit more prolonged use.

What physiological effects on the body does the use of tourniquets have?

- Increased production of xanthine oxidase which produces oxygen free radicals
- Increased cell to cell interactions and mediator cascades involving adhesion molecules
- Activation of the complement and coagulation cascades
- Hypercoagulability and increased plasma viscosity
- Endothelium damage

What are the potential complications with the use of tourniquets?

Local injuries:

- nerve injuries:
  - due to direct pressure beneath the cuff and shearing pressure at the cuff edge
  - associated with the function of peripheral nerves distal to the tourniquet and results in impairment of motor function and loss of vibration and position sense with sympathetic function and pain perception remaining unaffected
  - most frequently injured nerves are radial, ulnar, median and sciatic
  - injuries can range from paraesthesia to paralysis
- vascular injuries:
  - arterial spasm results from long periods of tourniquet ischaemia
  - thrombosis in atherosclerotic vessels
- muscle injuries:
  - occur beneath the cuff due to ischaemia and physical deformation
  - interstitial and intracellular oedema occurs within the muscle after tourniquet deflation, which can take several weeks to resolve

- compartment syndrome
- post-tourniquet syndrome
  - ischaemia-induced muscle injury causing myoglobinurea
  - ischaemia-induced oedema causes stiffness, muscle weakness and altered sensation in the area of tourniquet application
- skin injuries:
  - erythema or friction burns

Systemic injuries:
- cardio-respiratory effects:
  - tourniquet inflation results in elevation of the heart rate and blood pressure which may not be well tolerated in patients with poor cardiac function
  - tourniquet deflation is associated with a transient hypercapnia with a more pronounced effect seen in the lower limbs
- intracranial effects
  - significant rises in intracranial pressures are seen following tourniquet deflation in patients with severe head injuries
- metabolic effects:
  - release of lactate, myoglobin, K^+ and H^+ can cause acidosis
  - circulatory stasis and low oxygen concentrations can precipitate sickle cell crisis
- haematological effects:
  - tourniquet inflation can cause thrombo-embolism due to an increase in systemic hypercoagulability and plasma viscosity
  - tourniquet deflation is associated with a brief period of bleeding due to an increase in plasma thrombolytic activity
- increase in core body temperature

■ Transplantation

What do you understand by the terms orthoptic and heterotopic grafts?

Orthoptic graft: the graft is transplanted into the donor at the normal anatomical site, e.g. heart transplantation.

Heterotopic graft: the graft is transplanted into the donor at a location other than the normal anatomical site, e.g. renal transplantation.

What are the contraindications to transplantation?

Donor factors:
- hepatitis B, C and HIV infections
- active infection
- malignancy
- presence of significant systemic disease

Recipient factors:
- poor cardiovascular status
- presence of significant systemic disease
- presence of untreated infections (e.g. tuberculosis)
- age > 75 (relative contraindication)

What are the different types of graft rejection?

- Hyperacute (occurs immediately): antibody mediated; rare in modern days; irreversible
- Acute (occurs 5–14 days post transplantation): cell-mediated, usually reversible with corticosteroid treatment
- Chronic (occurs several months post transplantation): irreversible

What is the role of the major histocompatibility complex in transplantation?

The major histocompatibility complex (MHC) antigens are encoded for on chromosome 6 and are the most important antigens responsible for graft rejection. There are two classes of molecule encoded: class I antigens, which includes HLA-A, -B and -C and class II antigens, which include HLA-DR, HLA-DP and HLA-DQ. The most significant antigens to match in terms of graft survival are HLA-DR, HLA-B and HLA-A. The greater the number of matches, the less the chance of rejection.

List the complications of renal transplantation

Early:
- vascular:
  - haemorrhage
  - renal artery or vein thrombosis
- urological:
  - ureteric or bladder leak
  - ureteric reflux

Late:
- vascular:
  - renal artery stenosis
- urological:
  - ureteric stenosis
- cardiovascular:
  - hypertension
- malignancy:
  - Kaposi's sarcoma
  - lymphoma

What are the indications for cardiac, lung and liver transplantation?

Cardiac:
- congenital heart disease

- cardiomyopathies
- valvular heart disease
- amyloid disease

Lung:
- emphysema
- alpha-1 antitrypsin deficiency
- cystic fibrosis
- idiopathic pulmonary fibrosis

Liver:
- acute liver failure
- chronic liver disease
- liver tumours

List some commonly used immunosuppressant agents in transplantation surgery

- Corticosteroids
- Azathioprine
- Cyclosporins
- Tacrolimus
- Anti-IL-2 receptor antibodies (basiliximab and daclizumab)

■ Trauma I: Basic Principles

How would you manage a critically injured patient in the A&E department?

The trauma team constitutes a crucial approach to the early management of critically injured patients. These patients should be managed according to the ATLS® guidelines summarised below.

Airway and Cervical Spine control:

- clear airway: suction, chin lift, jaw thrust
- maintain airway: oropharyngeal, nasopharyngeal, endotracheal tube, needle or surgical cricothyroidectomy
- 100% oxygen at flow rate 15 l/min
- full cervical spine immobilisation: hard collar and lateral supports with straps across forehead and chin

Breathing:

- inspect neck and thorax
- determine respiratory rate
- auscultate for breath sounds

Circulation:

- shock assessment: skin colour, capillary refill, mental state, pulse, blood pressure, ECG, pulse oximetry
- control haemorrhage: direct pressure
- two large cannulas peripherally
- withdraw blood for FBC, U and E, glucose, X-match
- commence intravenous crystalloids
- give blood if necessary: full x-match, type specific, O Neg

Dysfunction (disability):

- pupils: size, equal, response to light
- conscious level: GCS, AVPU (Alert, Verbal stimuli, Pain stimuli, Unresponsive)

Exposure:
- remove all clothing
- prevent hypothermia: warm blankets; warm iv fluids

X-rays:
- lateral cervical spine: if clinically tender or non-tender but patient has distracting injuries or is unconscious. Assess for:
  - A – adequacy and alignment
  - B – bones: margins & architecture
  - C – cartilage/joints: joint spaces, surfaces
  - S – soft tissues: swelling, air in tissues (open wound/open fracture)
- chest (AP)
- pelvis

Secondary survey:
- examine patient head-to-toe
- log-roll: PR (and PV)
- insert tubes as necessary: urinary catheter, NGT, chest drain, central line, arterial line
- administer: anti-tetanus, antibiotics, analgesia

Obtain history: AMPLE
- Allergies
- Medications
- Past medical history
- Last meal
- Events of injury

Describe the Glasgow coma scale (GCS)

The GCS is scored between 3 and 15; 3 being the worst, and 15 the best. It is composed of three parameters: Best Eye Response, Best Verbal Response and Best Motor Response, as given below:
- Best Eye Response (4)
  1. No eye opening
  2. Eye opening to pain

3. Eye opening to verbal command
4. Eyes open spontaneously
- Best Verbal Response (5)
  1. No verbal response
  2. Incomprehensible sounds
  3. Inappropriate words
  4. Confused
  5. Orientated
- Best Motor Response (6)
  1. No motor response
  2. Extension to pain
  3. Flexion to pain
  4. Withdrawal from pain
  5. Localising pain
  6. Obeys commands

■ Trauma II: Head Injury

What do you understand by the terms primary and secondary head injuries?

Primary injury: insult caused to the brain at the time of impact. It is caused by shearing forces, which tear axonal tracts. The damage caused can be diffuse or focal. There is no treatment and the focus of intervention is to prevent secondary complications.

Secondary injury: occurs due to hypoxia (from obstructed airway or impaired respiratory drive), hypotension (from associated injuries) and raised intracranial pressure (due to haematoma, oedema, infection or abscess).

What is the initial management of the patient with a head injury?

Patients should be managed according to ATLS® principles:

- airway protection with C-spine immobilisation
- ensure adequacy of breathing
- maintain circulation and control haemorrhage
- assessment of the severity of head injury using the Glasgow Coma Score (GCS)

What are the indications for a CT scan?

- GCS <13 at any stage since injury or 2 h post-injury
- Focal neurological deficit
- Persistent confusion
- Any skull fracture
- Seizures following injury
- Amnesia

- Difficulty in assessing patient, e.g. due to alcohol
- Penetrating skull injury

What are the indications for a skull radiograph?
Same indications as for a CT, if scanning facilities are not available.

What are the criteria for admission following a head injury?
- Abnormality detected on CT scan
- Fluctuating GCS despite absence of abnormalities on a CT scan
- Patients on anticoagulant therapy

What are the indications for referral to a neurosurgeon?
- Presence of any intracranial bleeding
- GCS <8 despite adequate resuscitation
- Confusion >8 h post-injury
- Progressive neurological deficit
- Compound skull fractures
- A child with a tense fontanelle

What are the indications for intubation?
- GCS ≤ 8
- GCS 9–12 and patient is being transferred to another centre
- Uncontrolled seizures
- Loss of cough or gag reflex
- Respiratory compromise

What are the criteria for intracranial pressure monitoring?
- Head injury induced coma
- Patients with severe head injuries who require surgery for associated injuries

- Patients who require prolonged ventilation for pulmonary injuries

What are the risks of an intracranial haematoma in patients with head injuries?

- No skull fracture:
  - patient orientated   1:6000
  - patient not orientated   1:120
- Skull fracture:
  - patient orientated   1:32
  - patient not orientated   1:4

What are the possible complications following a head injury?

- Epilepsy
- Meningitis and cerebral abscesses
- Amnesia
- Post-concussional syndrome (headache, dizziness, poor concentration, memory impairment, behavioural changes)
- Chronic subdural haematoma
- Hydrocephalus
- Peptic ulceration
- Diabetes incipidus/SIADH
- Disseminated intravascular coagulation
- Encephalopathy (mainly in repeated head injuries, e.g. in boxers)

■ Trauma III: Abdominal Injury

How can abdominal injuries be classified?
By the mechanism of injury:
- blunt trauma:
  - direct blow, e.g. contact with steering wheel
  - shearing, e.g. seat belt injuries
  - deceleration: caused by differential movement of fixed and non-fixed body structures
- penetrating trauma:
  - low velocity, e.g. stab wounds
  - high velocity, e.g. rifle shots

How would you assess and manage a patient with an acute abdominal injury?
- History
  - RTA: type/speed of car, air bags, seat belt, type of impact
  - penetrating injury: type of weapon, distance from assault
- Examination:
  - inspection: abrasions, contusions, lacerations
  - palpation: guarding, rebound tenderness
  - percussion: tympanic (gastric dilatation); dull (haemoperitoneum)
  - auscultation: loss of bowel sounds
  - perineal examination: blood at urethral meatus, scrotal haematoma, bruising
  - PR: sphincter tone, prostate position, pelvic fracture, bleeding
  - PV: laceration, pelvic fracture
- Exploration of wound: to determine depth

- NG tube: reduces risk of aspiration and decompresses stomach
- Urinary catheter: if urinary tract injury suspected only catheterise after performing urethrography, cystography or IVP
- Evaluation of free intraperitoneal fluid: FAST, DPL, CT
- Laparotomy: if indicated on clinical grounds or after positive DPL/ imaging

What is FAST?

Focused Assessment with Sonography for Trauma (FAST) is a limited ultrasound examination directed solely at identifying the presence of free intraperitoneal or pericardial fluid. FAST examines four areas for free fluid: perihepatic and hepato-renal space; perisplenic area; pelvis and pericardium. It is indicated in the patient with blunt abdominal trauma who may or may not be haemodynamically unstable. FAST is poor at identifying and grading solid organ injury, bowel injury and retroperitoneal trauma. The average time to perform a FAST in the hands of an experienced operator is 2–3 mins. As a decision-making tool for identifying the need for laparotomy in hypotensive patients (Systolic BP <90), FAST has a sensitivity of 100% and specificity of 96%. It is less good at detecting solid organ injury with sensitivities ranging from 44 to 91%.

What are the advantages and disadvantages of USS, DPL and CT in abdominal trauma?

	USS	CT	DPL
Rapid	++		+
Portable	++		+
Non-invasive	++	++	
Operator dependent		++	++

(cont.)

	USS	CT	DPL
Sensitivity			+
Specificity	+	++	
Quantitative	+	++	
Cost	++		
Injury localisation	+	++	
Evaluation of retroperitoneum		++	
Evaluation of pericardium	++	+	
Ease of interpretation	+		++

++: Significant advantage.

+: Some advantage.

Briefly describe how you would perform a DPL

- Ensure patient has NGT and urinary catheter in situ
- Abdominal skin is prepared with betadine solution and LA injected
- Vertical midline sub-umbilical incision (1/3 distance between umbilicus and symphysis pubis)
- Linea alba divided; peritoneal cavity entered
- Aspirate contents of peritoneal cavity; if gross blood not obtained infuse warm saline and allow the fluid to remain for 5 min before draining
- Send 20 ml of aspirated/drained fluid for analysis
- Positive result if:
  - $>100\,000$ RBCs/mm^3
  - >500 WBCs/mm^3
  - aspirated fluid contains GI contents (food, faeces, bile) or bacteria

What are the indications for a laparotomy?

- Penetrating injury traversing the peritoneal cavity or associated with hypotension

- Blunt trauma with positive FAST, DPL or CT
- Blunt trauma with haemodynamic instability despite fluid resuscitation
- Peritonitis
- CXR: free air or retroperitoneal air

Trauma IV: Spinal Injury

How can spinal injuries be classified?

- Stable injuries: vertebral components won't be displaced by normal movement; loss of <50% of vertebral height
- Unstable injuries: further displacement of the injury may occur with movement; loss of ≥ 50% of vertebral height; angulation of thoracolumbar junction of > 20 degrees

What are the mechanisms of injury resulting in spinal trauma?

- Axial compression, e.g. burst fractures
- Hyperextension: common in the cervical spine
- Flexion
- Flexion with posterior distraction
- Flexion with rotation: causes dislocation with or without fractures
- Shearing

What is the management of patients with suspected acute spinal injuries?

- Obtain detailed history: mechanism of injury, neurological symptoms
- ABC with cervical spine immobilisation as per ATLS® protocol
- Prevent further damage: lie flat, log roll
- Examination: bruising, step, tenderness, neurological assessment

- X-rays: C-spine (AP and lateral including C7/T1); open mouth view of odontoid; AP and lateral view of other tender areas of spine
- Consider CT (to assess for bony injury) or MRI (to assess for soft tissue involvement)
- If neurological damage detected: discuss with the spinal team regarding administration of high dose methylprednisolone (use is controversial and needs to be given within 8 h of injury)
- Transfer to specialist unit if there is cord compression with progression of symptoms or for unstable fractures that need stabilisation
- For stable spinal injuries: analgesia, collar/brace/cast/ (burst fractures may benefit from operative stabilisation)

What are the potential complications of spinal injury?
- Neurological damage
- Deformity
- Chronic pain
- Respiratory tract infections: risk minimised by treating with early physiotherapy, ventilatory support, tracheostomy and suction, bronchoscopy
- DVT: anticoagulation therapy
- Malnutrition: early nutrition
- GI bleed secondary to stress ulceration: treat with antacids/ H_2 antagonists
- Urinary tract infections: prevented with bladder drainage, bladder retraining
- Pressure sores: turn every 2 h; early removal of spinal board
- Joint contractures: limb physiotherapy for passive movements +/− splintage
- Psychological: counselling

Describe the main types of incomplete cord injuries

Syndrome	Cause	Clinical features	Prognosis
Brown Sequard	Hemisection of cord	Loss of ipsilateral motor function, vibration and position sense; contralateral loss of pain and temperature	Good
Anterior cord	Cord infarction in territory supplied by anterior spinal artery	Motor loss; dorsal columns spared	Poor
Central cord	Vascular damage of cord in distribution of anterior spinal artery	Affects upper limbs more than lower limbs; motor and sensory loss	Fair

Define neurogenic and spinal shock

Neurogenic shock is the result of impairment of the descending sympathetic pathways within the spinal cord which causes a loss of vasomotor tone (hypotension) and loss of sympathetic innervation to the heart (bradycardia). This does not respond to fluid resuscitation (which can cause overload) and requires vasopressors and/or atropine.

Spinal shock is the flaccidity and loss of reflexes observed after spinal cord injury. The shock to the damaged cord may make it appear functionless even though not all areas are destroyed. The duration of this state can be variable.

■ Trauma V: Splenic Injury

How can splenic injuries be graded?
- Grade I
  - subcapsular haematoma <10% of surface area
  - capsular tear <1 cm in depth
- Grade II
  - subcapsular haematoma of 10–50% of surface area
  - intraparenchymal haematoma <5 cm in diameter
  - laceration of 1–3 cm in depth and not involving trabecular vessels
- Grade III
  - subcapsular haematoma >50% of surface area or expanding
  - intraparenchymal haematoma >5 cm or expanding
  - laceration >3 cm in depth or involving trabecular vessels
- Grade IV: laceration involving segmental or hilar vessels with devascularization >25% of the spleen
- Grade V: shattered spleen or hilar vascular injury

Which investigations may be useful in the diagnosis of splenic rupture?
- X-ray: left lower rib fractures, left hemidiaphragm elevation, left lower lobe atelectasis, pleural effusion, medial displacement of gastric bubble and inferior displacement of splenic flexure gas pattern
- FAST: fluid in the peritoneal cavity
- CT (with contrast): structural evaluation of spleen and surrounding organs

- Angiography: usually performed after CT; is less of a diagnostic modality and more of a preparation for therapeutic control of active bleeding sites
- DPL: rapidly determines if intraperitoneal blood is present

What are the management options in splenic trauma?
- Conservative: if haemodynamically stable; Hb stable for 48 h, minimal transfusion requirements ($\leq$2U), and grade 1 or 2 injuries. Patients should be monitored in HDU with immobilisation for 72 h
- Angio-embolisation: if splenic injury diagnosed with CT and evidence of ongoing bleed in a stable/stabilised patient
- Surgery: involves splenic repair or splenectomy. Indicated in patients who are haemodynamically unstable or have a continuing bleed not controlled with embolisation

What are the other indications for a splenectomy?
- Spontaneous rupture
- Hypersplenism
- Hereditary spherocytosis or elliptocytosis
- Idiopathic thrombocytopenic purpura
- Neoplasia
- Cysts: splenic, hydatid

What are the complications of splenectomy?
- Overwhelming post-splenectomy infection (OPSI): infection due to encapsulated bacteria (e.g. *Strep. pneumoniae, Haemophilus influenzae, Neisseria meningitides*); associated with a high mortality rate with the greatest risk in the first 2 years post-surgery.
- Prevention of OPSI: prophylactic immunisation: given 2 weeks prior to elective surgery and immediately post-surgery in emergency cases:

- Pneumococcal immunisation: reimmunise every 5 years
- Hib immunisation: reimmunise every 10 years
- Meningococcal immunisation: reimmunise every 5 years (plain A/C vaccine)
- Influenza immunisation: recommended yearly
- antibiotic prophylaxis: penicillin or amoxicillin required in children up to 16 years; in adults for the first 2 years after surgery and lifelong for invasive medical procedures and dental work
- Thrombocytosis: immediately following splenectomy, the platelet count rises and there is a greater risk of DVT and PE
- Gastric dilatation: occurs due to gastric ileus; pre-operatively a NGT should be placed and aspirated post surgery

■ Trauma VI: Thoracic Injury

What are the most common life-threatening chest injuries?

- Tension pneumothorax: airflow is unidirectional on inspiration but cannot escape during expiration due to one-way valve. Clinical features include: chest pain, air hunger, respiratory distress, shock, neck vein distention, cyanosis, tracheal deviation (opposite side), hyper-resonance and reduced breath sounds. Immediate decompression by inserting a large bore needle into the second ICS in the mid-clavicular line. Definitive treatment requires a chest drain
- Open pneumothorax: chest wall injury causes direct communication between inner thoracic cavity and external environment causing a pneumothorax. Immediate management includes closing the defect with sterile dressing that overlaps the wound edges thus providing a flutter type valve effect followed by chest drain insertion. Surgical closure of wound when patient stable
- Flail chest: segment of chest wall loses bony continuity with rest of the thoracic cage; associated with multiple rib fractures. There is paradoxical movement on respiration resulting in reduced tidal volume and ventilation. Management: analgesia, humidified O_2, ventilation $\pm$ intubation and chest drain
- Massive haemothorax: loss of > 1500 ml of blood into chest cavity or intercostal drain. The only indication when iv lines must be placed before insertion of a chest drain as sudden decompression of massive haemothorax may cause haemodynamic instability

- Cardiac tamponade: accumulation of pericardial fluid →
  ↑intrapericardial pressure → heart cannot fill → pumping
  stops. Clinical signs include Beck's triad (↑JVP, ↓BP, muffled
  heart sounds), JVP rises on inspiration (Kussmaul's sign) and
  pulsus paradoxus. Immediate pericardiocentesis is required.
  Thoracotomy not advised in A and E

Briefly describe how you would insert an intercostal chest drain

- Identify fifth intercostal space (nipple level) anterior to the
  mid-axillary line
- Infiltrate local anaesthetic down to pleura
- Small incision in the line of the rib
- Blunt dissection 'above the rib below'
- Puncture pleura with a clamp followed by finger sweep to
  clear clots or debris
- Pass large drain and connect to an underwater drain
- Pursestring suture to hold drain in place
- CXR to confirm position
- Maintain drain at level below the patient; clamp when
  moving the patient

▓ Urological Investigations I

Which investigations may be useful when assessing for urological pathology?

Urine testing:

- dipstick testing for:
  - blood cells: infection, calculus, bleeding from a tumour
  - leukocytes: infection, inflammation
  - protein: infection, inflammation, intrinsic renal pathology
  - nitrites: infection
  - glucose: diabetes mellitus
- microscopy: should be performed on a midstream specimen or a clean catch sample in children; results may show:
  - bacteria: significant growth is $\geq 10^5$ organisms/ml
  - red blood cells: haematuria
  - leukocytes: infection, inflammation, calculi, interstitial renal disease
  - casts: suggestive of renal disease
  - crystals: oxalate, cystine and phosphate in stone formers
- cytology: if tumour suspected
- 24 h collection: to measure creatinine clearance (can calculate GFR from this)

Blood:

- FBC:
  - leukocytosis: infections or malignancy
  - anaemia: chronic renal failure or malignancy
  - polycythaemia: renal cell carcinoma
- clotting: coagulopathies can cause haematuria
- creatinine and electrolytes:

- creatinine is a reliable indicator of renal filtration and function
- hyperkalaemia: acute renal failure
- hypercalcaemia in renal cell carcinoma (release of PTH-like hormone)
- PSA: used to detect and monitor prostate cancers

Plain radiographs (kidney, ureter, bladder (KUB)): have a limited use but may show:

- urinary stones: up to 90% are radio-opaque
- calcification of kidney, bladder or blood vessels

Ultrasound:

- transabdominal USS has now become the initial investigation for suspected renal, ureteric and testicular pathology. For kidneys it can assess renal size, show any masses or calculi and identify hydronephrosis. In the bladder, filling wall defects, wall thickness, calculi or tumours can be assessed. Scrotal USS is used to identify solid from cystic masses and guide needle biopsies for suspected masses
- transrectal USS is used to estimate prostate volume and allows guided biopsies to be taken

CT: can be performed with or without contrast and is used for:

- staging of urological malignancies
- assessing renal vasculature prior to partial nephrectomy
- diagnosing urolithiasis
- evaluation of renal trauma
- guiding needle biopsies of suspicious masses
- drain cysts/abscesses

MRI:

- better than CT at imaging the prostate
- used for investigating urological malignancies
- magnetic resonance urography and angiography are safer than the conventional procedures

Contrast studies:

- IVU: delineates the anatomy of the kidney outlines and collecting systems as well as providing dynamic and static information about the sites and possible causes of obstruction within the urinary tract. Disadvantages are that it is an invasive procedure, uses radiation, can miss renal masses and cannot be used in patients with renal failure or poor renal function
- retrograde ureterogram: contrast media is introduced retrogradely through a ureteric catheter inserted cystoscopically; performed if IVU has been unsatisfactory, other imaging modalities are unavailable or intraoperatively to assess for iatrogenic ureteric injury
- urethrogram: particularly useful in assessing urethral trauma but also used to evaluate strictures or posterior urethral valves
- micturating cystogram: contrast is introduced into the bladder and radiographs taken during voiding; allows assessment of ureteric reflux or fistulas

Radioisotope used to assess for:

- renal function
- obstruction
- bony metastases (technetium 99)

Angiography: used to assess for:

- circulation within tumours
- renal vasculature prior to partial nephrectomy
- vasculature anomalies: renal artery stenosis, AV malformation
- bleeding in renal trauma

Urodynamics: this is a dynamic assessment of function:

- urine flow test: provides an objective measurement of urine flow; reduced flow may indicate outflow obstruction or poor detrusor muscle contraction

- cystometrogram: used to differentiate between stress and urge incontinence

Endoscopy:

- flexible urethrocystoscopy: first line of investigation for most urethral and bladder pathologies, e.g. recurrent UTIs and haematuria
- ureteroscopy and renoscopy: performed under a general anaesthetic and allows direct visualisation and for biopsies to be taken

■ Urological Investigations II: Common Urological Conditions

Which investigations may be useful in the management of haematuria, urinary stone disease, urinary tract infections, outflow obstruction and incontinence?

Investigation	Condition				
	Haematuria	Urinary stone disease	Urinary tract infections	Outflow obstruction	Incontinence
Urine testing	Infection; cytology to exclude tumour	24 h collection of Ca, PO_4^-, oxalate, urate	Leukocytes, nitrites, protein, blood, bacteria	Microscopy + culture: haematuria or infection	To exclude infection
Blood tests	Hb to assess severity U and E: renal function PSA: in men	Serum Ca^{2+} WCC if infection U and E: renal function	↑ WCC U and EC cultures (if toxic)	FBC: assess severity or infection U and E: renal function	U and E: renal function
KUB	Performed with IVU/USS	90% radio-opaque	For pyelo-nephritis	Assess for calculi	
USS	Assess for renal mass but ureteric lesions will be missed	Renal USS: for radiolucent stones or if percutaneous nephrostomy needed for obstruction	Renal USS: for recurrent lower tract infections in women; males after first infection	Bladder: measure post-micturition residual volume; renal USS for hydro-nephrosis; Transrectal: if cause is? prostate cancer	Bladder USS: shows if bladder fails to empty on voiding

(cont.)

Investigation	Condition				
	Haematuria	Urinary stone disease	Urinary tract infections	Outflow obstruction	Incontinence
CT		If allergic to contrast			
Contrast studies	IVU to assess collecting system and ureter	IVU will confirm location of stones; if obstruction suspected	IVU if USS suggests anatomical abnormality	Urethrogram: for strictures or posterior urethral valves	
Radioisotope scan		If obstruction present	If PUJ obstruction suspected	Determines degree of obstruction	
Urodynamics				Flow rate test	Cystometrogram/video urodynamics
Endoscopy	All patients must have a cystoscopy		Cystoscopy for recurrent patients		

■ Wound Classification

How can wounds be classified?

- By cause:
  - traumatic (sharp or blunt)
  - iatrogenic (following surgery)
  - burns (thermal, electrical or chemical)
- Length of time since formation:
  - acute (<6 weeks old)
  - chronic (>6 weeks old)
- By depth:
  - superficial: do not traverse the subdermis layer of skin
  - deep: traverse the subdermis layer
- By site, e.g. midline laparotomy, Lanz, suprapubic, thoracotomy
- By complexity:
  - simple: involves skin and subcutaneous tissues without significant tissue loss
  - complex: significant tissue loss or devitalisation; communicates with deeper structures, e.g. internal organs or joints
  - complicated: wounds with superimposed complication, i.e. infection, haematoma, ischaemia or compartment syndrome
- By mode of injury:
  - abrasion (only involves the outer layers of the skin)
  - ulceration (defect in the epithelial lining)
  - incision (wounds caused by sharp objects)
  - laceration (wounds caused by blunt objects)
  - degloving injury (laceration in which skin is sheared from underlying fascia)

- By degree of contamination:
  - clean
  - clean-contaminated
  - contaminated
  - dirty

What are the infection rates in wounds classified by degree of contamination?

Wound type	Example	Approximate infection rate (%)
Clean	Incision through non-inflamed tissue; no entry into the GU or GI tract	<2
Clean-contaminated	Entry into hollow viscus other than colon; minimal controlled contamination	8–10
Contaminated	Breaching of hollow viscus with spillage; opening of colon; open fractures; penetrating bites	1–20
Dirty	Gross pus; perforated viscus or traumatic wounds left open for >4 h	>25

■ Wound Healing

Describe the different phases of wound healing

- Coagulation: mast cell activation results in release of cytokines with local vasoconstriction and migration of intravascular cells into the extravascular space within the wound area. A haemostatic clot results from platelets and fibrin
- Epithelialisation: after the blood clot forms, epithelial cells close to the cut edge as well as stem cells from the basal part of the epithelium and adjacent pilosebaceous follicles migrate over viable tissue beneath the surface blood clot. For wound healing by primary intention, the wound may be bridged by epithelium within 48 hours which then rapidly stratifies
- Organisation: neutrophils attracted by cytokines initiate an acute inflammatory process within 24 hours. This is followed by an influx of macrophages accompanied by a proliferation of fibroblasts and in-growth of new blood vessels. Through the release of cytokines, e.g. PDGF, TGF-alpha and EGF, these inflammatory cells regulate connective tissue matrix repair. In wounds that heal by secondary intention, this matrix of proliferating fragile capillary buds, fibroblasts and macrophages is known as granulation tissue
- Collagen synthesis and remodelling: collagen synthesis by fibroblasts peaks about 5 days after injury when Type 3 collagen predominates. Vitamin C deficiency or hypoxia will compromise intracellular synthesis and result in insufficient wound strength. The finished collagen molecule consists of three polypeptide chains. Once it reaches the extracellular environment, collagen cross-linking occurs to form fibrils

and fibres of collagen. After 7 days, collagen synthesis gradually declines and remodelling occurs. Remodelling refers to the equilibrium between collagen synthesis and degradation. As old fibres are broken down, new fibres are synthesised with increasing density of cross-links. The tensile strength of the wound increases over months by replacement of some Type 3 collagen by Type 1 collagen, and remodelling in response to mechanical stress

- Wound maturation: some of the fibroblasts involved in healing contain myofibrils, which have contractile properties and play a role in the contraction of wounds. Sensory nerve fibres may grow into the scar in about 3 weeks but specialised nerve endings such as Pacinian corpuscles do not reform. The initial scar is usually red and raised due to underlying proliferative processes and vascularity. The blood vessels gradually decrease in number resulting in a pale scar

Define wound closure by primary, secondary and tertiary intentions

- In primary intention, wound edges are approximated using sutures, steri-strips or staples. Healing occurs with minimal fibrosis and tissue loss
- In secondary intention, wound edges are not apposed and healing occurs by granulation tissue filling the gap. This is associated with extensive fibrosis
- In tertiary intention, the wound is closed several days after its formation

Why might wounds be left to heal by secondary intention?

- When there is extensive loss of epithelium and wound closure by primary intention is not possible
- If the wound is contaminated or infected

- When the wound was initially closed by primary intention but has subsequently broken down
- Closure of the wound is possible but would not be tension free
- Closure of the wound would result in a tight compartment

What is granulation tissue?

It is temporary tissue that is formed during wound healing by secondary intention. It comprises extracellular matrix (collagens, proteoglycans, fibronectin, laminin); specialised cells (fibroblasts, macrophages, endothelial cells); and a rich network of capillary vessels. Granulation tissue is eventually remodelled and replaced by scar tissue.

What do the terms wound dehiscence and evisceration mean?

Dehiscence: partial or total disruption of any or all of the layers of an operative wound.
Evisceration: rupture of all the layers of the abdominal wall with extrusion of the abdominal viscera.

How are they treated?

Both are normally caused due to poor surgical technique in wound closure or due to infection. They usually manifest in the second post-operative week. Management includes analgesia, fluid resuscitation, sterile wound dressing and re-suturing under general anaesthesia.

What are the predisposing factors for wound break down?

- Local factors:
  - wound infection
  - site of wound
  - inadequate closure

- poor blood supply
- wound haematoma
- minimal foreign material
- excessive movement
- General factors:
  - elderly patients
  - diabetes mellitus
  - malnutrition
  - corticosteroids
  - obesity
  - malignancy
  - ionising radiation
  - renal failure
  - immunodeficiency
- Nutritional factors:
  - vitamins A, B6 and C deficiency
  - zinc deficiency
  - copper deficiency
  - protein deficiency